Understanding Patient Safety

Understanding Patient Safety

Robert M. Wachter, MD
Professor and Associate Chairman,
Department of Medicine
Marc and Lynne Benioff Endowed Chair
Chief of the Division of Hospital Medicine
University of California, San Francisco
Chief of the Medical Service
Chair of the Patient Safety Committee,
UCSF Medical Center
San Francisco, California

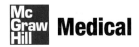

*New York Chicago San Francisco Lisbon London Madrid
Mexico City Milan New Delhi San Juan Seoul
Singapore Sydney Toronto*

Understanding Patient Safety

2 3 4 5 6 7 8 9 0   DOC/DOC   0 9 8

ISBN 978-0-07-148277-6
MHID 0-07-148277-6

This book was set in Times by International Typesetting and Composition.
The editors were Jim Shanahan and Karen Edmanson.
The production supervisor was Thomas Kowalczyk.
Project management was provided by International Typesetting and Composition.
The index was prepared by Kevin Broccoli.
RR Donnelley/Crawfordsville was printer and binder.

This book is printed on acid-free paper.

Cataloging-in-Publication Data for this title is on file with the Library of Congress.

Contents

CHAPTER SEVEN
Human Factors and
Errors at the Person-Machine Interface **75**

CHAPTER EIGHT
Transition and Handoff Errors. **85**

CHAPTER NINE
Teamwork and Communication Errors **99**

CHAPTER TEN
Nosocomial Infections **109**

Preface

In late 1999, the U.S. Institute of Medicine published *To Err is Human: Building a Safer Health Care System.*[1] Although the IOM has published more than 300 reports since *To Err*, none have been nearly as influential. The reason: extrapolating from data from the Harvard Medical Practice Study,[2,3] performed a decade earlier, the authors came up with the estimate that 44,000–98,000 Americans die each year from medical errors. More shockingly, they translated these numbers into the now-famous "jumbo jet units," pointing out that this death toll would be the equivalent of a jumbo jet crashing each and every day in the United States.

Although some critiqued the jumbo jet analogy as hyperbolic, I like it for several reasons. First, it provides a vivid and tangible icon for the magnitude of the problem (obviously, if extended to the rest of the world, the toll would be many times higher). Secondly, if in fact a jumbo jet was crashing every day, who among us would even consider flying electively! Third, and most importantly, consider for a moment what our society would be doing and spending to fix the problem if there were a jumbo jet (or even merely a regional commuter plane) crashing every day. The answer, of course, is that there would be no limit to what we would do to fix *that* problem. Yet prior to the IOM Report, we were doing next to nothing to make patients safer.

This is not to imply for a moment that the millions of committed, hard working, and well-trained doctors, nurses, pharmacists, therapists, and healthcare administrators *wanted* to harm people from medical mistakes. They did not—to the degree that Albert Wu has labeled providers who commit an error that causes terrible harm "second victims."[4] Yet we now understand that the problem of medical errors is not fundamentally one of "bad apples" (though there are certainly some), but rather one of competent providers working in a chaotic system that has not prioritized safety. As my colleague Kaveh Shojania and I wrote in our book, *Internal Bleeding*:

> Decades of research, mostly from outside healthcare, has confirmed our own medical experience: Most errors are made by good but fallible people working in dysfunctional systems, which means that making care safer depends on buttressing the system to prevent or catch the inevitable lapses of mortals. This logical approach is common in other complex, high-tech industries, but it has been woefully ignored in medicine. Instead, we have steadfastly clung to the view that an error is a moral failure by an individual, a posture that has left patients feeling angry and ready to blame, and providers feeling guilty and demoralized. Most importantly, it hasn't done a damn thing to make healthcare safer.[5]

Try for a moment to think of systems in healthcare that were truly "hardwired" for safety prior to 1999. Can you come up with any? I can only think of one: the double-checking that nurses did before releasing a unit of blood to prevent ABO transfusion errors. Now think about other error-prone areas: preventing harmful drug interactions or giving patients medicines to which they are allergic; ensuring that patients' preferences regarding resuscitation are respected; guaranteeing that the correct limbs are operated on; making sure primary care doctors have the necessary information after a hospitalization; diagnosing patients with chest pain in the emergency department correctly—none of these were organized in ways that could ensure safety.

Interestingly, many of the answers were there for the taking, from industries as diverse as take-out restaurants to nuclear power plants, from commercial aviation to automobile manufacturing. I have called the process of taking the insights from other industries and applying them to healthcare "translocational research,"[6] and there are now dozens of examples of successes (Table P-1). Why does healthcare depend so much on the experiences of other industries to improve safety? In part, it is because other industries have long recognized the diverse expertise that must be tapped to produce the best possible product at the lowest cost. In healthcare, the absence of any incentive to focus on quality and safety, our burgeoning biomedical knowledge base, our siloed approach to professional training, and, frankly, professional hubris, have caused us to

TABLE P-1

Examples of "translocational" research in patient safety

Strategy (Described in Chapter XX)	Non-Healthcare Example	Study Demonstrating Value in Healthcare	Impetus for Wider Implementation in Healthcare
Improved ratios of providers to "customers" (Chapter 16)	Teacher-to-student ratios (such as in class-size initiatives)	Aiken (2002)	California legislation mandating minimum nurse-to-patient ratios, other pressure
Decrease provider fatigue (Chapter 16)	Consecutive work-hour limitations for pilots, truck drivers	Landrigan (2004)	Accreditation Council for Graduate Medical Education (ACGME) regulations limiting resident duty hours
Improve teamwork and communication (Chapter 15)	Crew Resource Management (CRM) in aviation	Morey (2002)	None yet for healthcare CRM, but on the horizon if evidence becomes more robust
Use of simulators (Chapter 17)	Simulator use in aviation and the military	Sutherland (2006)	Medical simulation now required for credentialing for certain procedures, growing interest
Executive Walk Rounds (Chapter 22)	"Management by Walking Around" in business	Frankel (2003)	Executive Walk Rounds not required, but increasingly popular practice
Bar coding (Chapter 13)	Use of bar coding in manufacturing, retail, and food sales	Poon (2006)	U.S. Food and Drug Administration now requires bar codes on most prescription medications; bar coding (or radiofrequency identification) may ultimately be required in many identification processes

Reproduced with permission from Wachter RM. Playing well with others: "translocational research" in patient safety. AHRQ WebM&M (serial online), September 2005. Available at: http://webmm.ahrq.gov/perspective.aspx?perspectiveID=9.

Aiken LH, Clarke SP, Sloane DM, et al. Hospital nurse staffing and patient mortality, nurse burnout, and job dissatisfaction. *JAMA* 2002;288:1987–1993.

Frankel A, Graydon-Baker E, Neppl C, et al. Patient safety leadership walkrounds. *Jt Comm J Qual Improv* 2003;29:16–26.

Landrigan CP, Rothschild JM, Cronin JW, et al. Effect of reducing interns' work hours on serious medical errors in intensive care units. *N Engl J Med* 2004;351:1838–1848.

Morey JC, Simon R, Jay GD, et al. Error reduction and performance improvement in the emergency department through formal teamwork training: evaluation results of the MedTeams project. *Health Serv Res* 2002;37:1553–1581.

Poon EG, Cina JL, Churchill W, et al. Medication dispensing errors and potential adverse drug events before and after implementing bar code technology in the pharmacy. *Ann Intern Med* 2006;145:426–434.

Sutherland LM, Middleton PF, Anthony A. Surgical simulation: a systematic review. *Ann Surg* 2006;243:291–300.

look inward, not outward, for answers. The fact that we are now routinely seeking insights from aviation, manufacturing, education, and other industries, and embracing paradigms from engineering, sociology, psychology, and management, may prove to be the most enduring benefit of the patient safety movement.

All of this is what makes the field of patient safety so exciting. To keep patients safe will take a uniquely interdisciplinary effort, one in which doctors, nurses, pharmacists, and administrators forge new types of relationships. It will require that we tamp down our traditional rigid hierarchies, without forgetting the importance of leadership or compromising crucial lines of authority. It will involve new resources, even as we recognize that investments in safety may well pay off in new efficiencies, lower provider turnover, and fewer expensive complications to clean up. It will require a thoughtful embrace of this new notion of systems thinking, while recognizing the absolute importance of the well-trained and committed caregiver. Again, from *Internal Bleeding*:

> Although there is much we can learn from industries that have long embraced the systems approach . . . medical care is much more complex and customized than flying an Airbus: At 3 A.M., the critically ill patient needs superb and compassionate doctors and nurses more than she needs a better checklist. We take seriously the awesome privileges and responsibilities that society grants us as physicians, and don't believe for a second that individual excellence and professional passion will become expendable even after our trapeze swings over netting called a "safer system." In the end, medical errors are a hard enough nut to crack that we need excellent doctors *and* safer systems.[5]

This book aims to teach the key principles of patient safety to a diverse audience: physicians, nurses, pharmacists, other healthcare providers, quality and safety professionals, risk managers, hospital administrators, and others. It is suitable for all levels of readers: from the senior physician trying to learn this new way of approaching his or her work, to the medical or nursing student, to the risk manager being asked to get more involved in institutional safety efforts. The fact that the same book can speak to all of these groups (whereas few clinical textbooks could) is another mark of the interdisciplinary nature of this field. Although many of the examples and references will be from the United States (mostly because they are more familiar to me), my travels and studies have convinced me that most of the issues are the same internationally, and that all countries can learn much from each other. I have made every effort, therefore, to make the book relevant to a geographically diverse audience, and have included key references and tools from outside the United States.

The book is divided into three main sections. In the introduction, I'll describe the epidemiology of error, distinguish safety from quality, and discuss the key mental models that inform our modern understanding of the field of patient safety. In Section II, I'll review different error types, taking advantage of real cases to describe various kinds of mistakes and safety hazards, introduce new terminology, and discuss what we know about how errors happen and how they can be prevented. Although many prevention strategies will be touched on in Section II, more general issues regarding various strategies (both from individual institutional and broader policy perspectives) will be reviewed in Section III. After a concluding chapter, the Appendix includes a wide array of resources, from helpful web sites to a patient safety glossary. To keep the book a manageable size, my goal will be to be more useful and engaging than comprehensive—interested readers will find more thorough references (particularly for individual topic areas) throughout the text.

Some of the material for this book will be derived or adapted from other works that I've had the privilege to edit or write. Specifically, some of the case presentations will be drawn from *Internal Bleeding: The Truth Behind America's Terrifying Epidemic of Medical Mistakes*,[5] the "Quality Grand Rounds" series in the *Annals of Internal Medicine* (Appendix I), and AHRQ WebM&M.[7] I am particularly grateful to my partner in many of these efforts, Dr. Kaveh Shojania, now of the University of Ottawa, for his remarkable contributions to the safety field and for reviewing an earlier draft of this book and authoring the glossary. Thanks too to my other partners on Quality Grand Rounds (Dr. Sanjay Saint and Amy Markowitz), AHRQ WebM&M and AHRQ Patient Safety Network[8] (Drs. Brad Sharpe, Tracy Minichiello, Niraj Sehgal, Russ Cucina, and Sumant Ranji; Professors Mary Blegen and Brian Alldredge; and Lorri Zipperer, Erin Hartman, and Kristen Fitzhenry), and to the sponsoring organizations (Rugged Land, publisher of *Internal Bleeding*; the California HealthCare Foundation and the *Annals of Internal Medicine* for Quality Grand Rounds; and the U.S. Agency for Healthcare Research and Quality for AHRQ WebM&M and PSNet). Thanks too to Bryan Haughom, a talented UCSF medical student who coauthored Chapter 7 and helped research some of the other chapters, to my administrative assistant Mary Whitney, and to Jim Shanahan of McGraw-Hill, who conceived of this book and has nurtured it every step of the way. This book would not have been possible without the contributions of all these extraordinary people and organizations.

Finally, although this is not primarily a book written for patients, it is a book written *about* patients. As patient safety becomes professionalized (with "patient safety officers"), it will inevitably become jargonized— "We need a root cause analysis!" "What did the Failure Mode Effects Analysis show?"—and this evolution will make it easy to take our eyes off the ball. We now know that tens of thousands of people in the United States—and many times that around the world—die each year because of preventable medical errors. Moreover, every day millions of people check into hospitals or clinics worried that they'll be killed in the process of receiving chemotherapy, undergoing surgery, or delivering a baby. Our efforts must be focused on preventing these errors, and the associated anxiety that patients feel when they receive medical care in an unsafe, chaotic environment.

Some have argued that medical errors are the dark side of medical progress, an inevitable consequence of the ever-increasing complexity of modern medicine. Perhaps a few errors fit this description, but most do not. I can easily envision a system in which patients benefit from all the modern miracles available to us, and yet do so in reliable organizations that take advantage of all the necessary tools and systems to "get it right" the vast majority of the time. Looking back at the remarkable progress that has been made in the first decade since the publication of the Institute of Medicine report on medical errors, I am confident that we can create such a system. My hope is that this book makes a small contribution toward achieving that goal.

REFERENCES

1. Kohn L, Corrigan J, Donaldson M, eds. *To Err is Human: Building a Safer Health System.* Washington, DC: Committee on Quality of Health Care in America, Institute of Medicine: National Academy Press, 2000.
2. Brennan TA, Leape LL, Laird NM, et al. Incidence of adverse events and negligence in hospitalized patients. Results of the Harvard Medical Practice Study I. *N Engl J Med* 1991;324:370–376.
3. Leape LL, Brennan TA, Laird N, et al. The nature of adverse events and negligence in hospitalized patients. Results of the Harvard Medical Practice Study II. *N Engl J Med* 1991;324:377–384.
4. Wu AW. Medical error: the second victim. *West J Med* 2000;172:358–359.

5. Wachter RM, Shojania KG. *Internal Bleeding: The Truth Behind America's Terrifying Epidemic of Medical Mistakes*. New York, NY: Rugged Land, 2004.
6. Wachter RM. Playing well with others: "translocational research" in patient safety. AHRQ WebM&M (serial online), September 2005. Available at: http://webmm.ahrq.gov/perspective.aspx?perspectiveID=9.
7. Available at: http://webmm.ahrq.gov.
8. Available at: http://psnet.ahrq.gov.

An Introduction to Patient Safety and Medical Errors

CHAPTER ONE

The Nature and Frequency of Medical Errors and Adverse Events

ADVERSE EVENTS, PREVENTABLE ADVERSE EVENTS, AND ERRORS

Although Hippocrates said "first, do no harm" over 2000 years ago and many hospitals have long hosted conferences to discuss errors (Morbidity and Mortality, or "M&M," conferences), until recently medical errors were considered an inevitable by-product of modern medicine or the unfortunate detritus of bad providers. This began to change in late 1999, with the publication by the Institute of Medicine (IOM) of *To Err is Human: Building a Safer Health System*.[1] This report, which estimated that 44,000 to 98,000 Americans die each year from medical mistakes, generated tremendous public and media attention, and set the stage for unprecedented efforts to improve patient safety. Of course, these seminal works built on a rich tapestry of inquiry and leadership in the field of patient safety (Appendix III), familiar to a small, committed group of devotees but generally unknown to mainstream providers, administrators, policymakers, and patients.

The IOM death estimate, which was drawn from thousands of chart reviews in New York,[2,3] Colorado, and Utah[4] in the late 1980s and early 1990s, was followed by studies that showed huge numbers of medication errors, communication problems in intensive care units (ICU), gaps in the discharge process, retained sponges in the operating room—in short, everywhere one looked, one found evidence of major problems in patient safety. Moreover, accompanying this information in the professional literature were scores of dramatic reports in the lay media: errors involving the wrong patient going to a procedure or the wrong limb being operated on, chemotherapy overdoses, botched transplants, patients released from the emergency department (ED) to die later from their myocardial infarction or aortic dissection, and more (Table 1–1).

The patient safety literature contains many overlapping terms to describe safety-related issues. Although the terms sometimes confuse more than clarify, two key distinctions underlie most of the terminology and allow one to keep it relatively straight. First, because patients commonly experience adverse outcomes, it is important to distinguish adverse outcomes as a result of medical care from morbidity and mortality that patients suffer as a consequence of their underlying medical conditions— the former are known as *adverse events*, defined as any injury or harm resulting from medical care. Second, because patients may experience harm from their medical care in the absence of any errors (i.e., from accepted complications of surgery or medication side effects), the patient safety literature separates *preventable adverse events* from *nonpreventable* ones. Figure 1–1 shows a Venn diagram depicting these various terms.

Now, where do *errors* or *mistakes* fit in? The safety literature commonly defines an error as "an act of commission (doing something wrong) or omission (failing to do the right thing) leading to an undesirable outcome or significant potential for such an outcome."[5] Note that some errors do not result in adverse events (Figure 1–1)—we generally characterize these as "near misses." Note too that some errors involve care that falls below a professional standard of care—these are characterized as negligent and may create legal liability in some systems (Chapter 18). Finally, although most preventable adverse events involve errors, not all of them do (see "The Challenges of Measuring Errors and Safety," below). For this and other reasons, many safety experts prefer to highlight preventable adverse events (rather than errors) as the main target of the safety field, since this terminology does not necessarily imply that a specific provider was responsible for any harm, an implication that may generate defensiveness by caregivers or an inordinate focus by the organization on

TABLE 1-1

Selected medical errors that garnered extensive media attention in the United States

Error	Institution	Year	Impact
An 18-year-old woman, Libby Zion, daughter of a prominent reporter, dies of a medical mistake, partly due to lax resident supervision	Cornell's New York Hospital	1984	Public discussion regarding resident training, supervision, and work hours. Led to New York law regarding supervision and work hours, ultimately culminating in ACGME duty hour regulations (Chapter 16)
Betsy Lehman, a *Boston Globe* healthcare reporter, dies of a chemotherapy overdose	Harvard's Dana-Farber Cancer Institute	1994	New focus on medication errors, role of ambiguity in prescriptions and possible role of computerized prescribing and decision support (Chapters 4 and 13)
Willie King, a 51-year-old diabetic, has the wrong leg amputated	University Community Hospital, Tampa, Florida	1995	New focus on wrong-site surgery, ultimately leading to Joint Commission's Universal Protocol to prevent these errors (Chapter 5)
Two healthy young volunteers (Jesse Gelsinger and Ellen Roche) die while participating in research studies	University of Pennsylvania (JG); Johns Hopkins (ER)	1999 and 2001	New focus on protecting research subjects from harm
18-month-old Josie King dies of dehydration	Johns Hopkins Hospital	2001	Josie's parents form an alliance with Johns Hopkins' leadership (leading to the Josie King Foundation and catalyzing Hopkins' safety initiatives), demonstrating the power of institutional and patient collaboration
Jesica Santillan, a 17-year-old girl from Mexico, dies after receiving a heart-lung transplant of the wrong blood type	Duke University Medical Center	2003	New focus on errors in transplantation, and on enforcing strict, high reliability protocols for communication of crucial data (Chapter 2)

Abbreviation: ACGME, Accreditation Council for Graduate Medical Education.

5

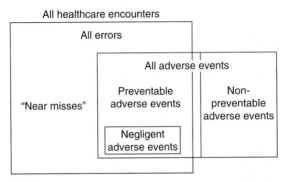

FIGURE 1–1. Venn diagram depicting patient safety terminology.

dealing with the individual rather than the system (Chapter 2). Others, however, feel that the terms "error" or "mistake" pack the visceral punch needed to catalyze change, while "preventable adverse events" seems too careful, perhaps even politically correct.

Whatever the terminology, these distinctions are important to understand as one tries to interpret the safety literature or individual cases. For example, a patient placed appropriately on warfarin for chronic atrial fibrillation who develops a gastrointestinal (GI) bleed while his or her international normalized ratio (INR) is therapeutic is the victim of an adverse event, but not a preventable adverse event or a medical error. If the patient had bled in the setting of a supratherapeutic INR, but there was no overt error on the part of the physician, the patient would be said to have suffered a preventable adverse event (but not an error). Finally, it would be a preventable adverse event *and an error* if the INR was supratherapeutic because the physician prescribed a new medication without checking for possible drug interactions.

Before leaving the (admittedly arcane) area of patient safety terminology, I should add that some safety experts bristle at the distinction between preventable and nonpreventable adverse events, arguing that some episodes of harm previously thought unpreventable are now known to be preventable with better systems. Some even contend that labeling such events "nonpreventable" is defeatist and self-fulfilling. Probably the best known examples supporting this argument are catheter-related bloodstream infections and ventilator-associated pneumonias, both once felt to be inevitable consequences of modern medicine but now known to be largely preventable with the consistent application of a variety of safety practices[6] (Chapter 10). Although this point of view has considerable merit, the distinction between preventability and nonpreventability permeates the literature, and blurring it risks a public perception that all adverse events result from errors, which they do not.

THE CHALLENGES OF MEASURING ERRORS AND SAFETY

At XYZ hospital, the patient safety officer has become concerned about the frequency of medication errors. One patient received a 10-fold overdose of insulin when the order "please give 10U regular insulin" was interpreted as "100 regular insulin." Another patient received a cephalosporin antibiotic for pneumonia, despite being allergic to this class of drugs. A third suffered a GI bleed when an overdose of warfarin led to over-anticoagulation.

In response to these incidents, the hospital is considering whether to invest in a computerized provider order entry system (CPOE) at a cost of 20 million dollars. The Chief Financial Officer (CFO), knowing that this expense will mean that the hospital will have to forego its planned purchase of a new 64-slice computed tomography (CT) scanner and the construction of two new operating rooms (investments with near-guaranteed positive returns on investment), asks the safety officer, "How will we know that we've made a difference?"

The CFO's question seems relatively straightforward, but is much harder to answer than you might think. Let's consider various ways of measuring errors.

The most common method is self-reports of errors by providers, usually referred to as *incident reports*. These reports have traditionally been completed by pencil and paper; they are increasingly being inputted through a computerized system. Incident reports (see also Chapter 14) might seem to be a reliable way of tracking errors, but there are several problems with using them to measure the frequency of errors. First, while nurses tend to report errors through incident reporting systems, few doctors do,[7] either not reporting at all or preferring to use informal channels (such as, in teaching programs, telling the chief residents). Secondly, since most reporting systems are voluntary, the frequency of reports will be influenced by many factors other than the number of errors. Let's say the institution has improved its safety culture (Chapter 15) recently, such that reporting of errors is now strongly encouraged by local leaders and incident reports result in tangible action. Moreover, a new user–friendly computerized incident reporting system has been rolled out. Under these circumstances, an increase in incident reports might well reflect the same number, or even fewer, errors being reported more assiduously. This conundrum distinguishes measuring patient safety from measuring the quality of care, which is less dependent on voluntary reporting and thus can be done more reliably (Chapter 3).

Given the problem in using incident reports to measure the frequency of errors, are there other ways? One could *review charts* for evidence of errors. This, in fact, is what the Harvard Medical Practice Study investigators did as they searched for "preventable adverse events."[2–4] Unfortunately, chart review is expensive and labor intensive (this burden may be eased somewhat by electronic medical record systems, particularly if they capture data in organized ways rather than as free text), poor charting may be on the same gene as the propensity to commit errors (thus penalizing institutions and providers who chart their care well), the medicolegal climate almost certainly induces some "buffing of the chart" when an error has occurred, and chart review is simply not a very reliable way to determine whether an error has occurred.[8] The latter problem is partly due to the inevitability of hindsight bias, in which knowledge of the final outcome influences the reviewer's determination regarding whether a given act was an error, a problem that also besets many malpractice investigations.[9]

Many institutions are using *trigger tools* to search for errors. The premise behind trigger tools is that some errors in care will engender a response that can be tracked.[10] For example, the patient with a warfarin overdose may be given a dose of Vitamin K or fresh frozen plasma to counteract the excess anticoagulant. A trigger tool looking for the administration of these antidotes would have identified the case.[11] Or a patient insufficiently observed on the medical ward may have an unexpected need to be transferred urgently to the ICU. While trigger tools are neither perfectly sensitive nor specific, they can often identify cases of medical errors that incident reporting systems miss. But because many triggers don't actually represent errors, they are best used as a screen, to be followed by more detailed chart review and discussion with the involved providers. Examples of commonly employed trigger tools can be found in Table 1–2.

Substantial recent research has focused on the identification of *patient safety indicators* gleaned from large administrative datasets. The most widely used indicator set is the Agency for Healthcare Research and

TABLE 1–2

Selected triggers from the Institute for Healthcare Improvement's (IHI) Global Trigger Tool

Care module triggers

Any code or arrest
Abrupt drop of >25% in hematocrit
Patient fall
Readmission within 30 days
Transfer to higher level of care

Surgical module triggers

Return to surgery
Intubation/reintubation in postanesthesia care unit
Intra- or postoperative death
Postoperative troponin level >1.5 ng/mL
Operative time >6 h

Medication module triggers

PTT > 100 s
INR > 6
Rising BUN or creatinine >2 times baseline
Vitamin K administration
Narcan (Naloxone) use
Abrupt medication stop

Intensive care module triggers

Pneumonia onset
Readmission to intensive care
Intubation/reintubation

Perinatal module

Apgar <7 at 5 min
3rd or 4th degree lacerations

ED module

Readmission to ED within 48 h
Time in ED >6 h

Abbreviations: PTT, partial thromboplastin time; BUN, blood urea nitrogen; ED, emergency department.
Reproduced with permission from Griffin FA, Resar RK. *IHI Global Trigger Tool for Measuring Adverse Events.* Cambridge, MA: Institute for Healthcare Improvement, 2007. (Available on www.IHI.org)

Quality's (AHRQ) Patient Safety Indicators (PSIs), which presently measure 27 outcomes or processes that are plausibly related to safety[12] (Appendix V). Although AHRQ cautions that these indicators should only be used as potential clues for problems (because their source is usually administrative data that may be unreliable and, like triggers, some indicators are not specific for errors), some commercial vendors do just that, and the media disseminate these (often sensational) findings widely.

A variety of other methods can be used to study errors and adverse events, and each has advantages and disadvantages[13] (Table 1–3). The key point is that frequency of errors and adverse events will vary markedly depending on the method used. For example, Leape found that, while voluntary self-reporting picks up only 1 of every 500 adverse drug events, a combination of chart review and computer screening caught 1 in 10.[14]

THE FREQUENCY AND IMPACT OF ERRORS

In part because of different definitions and assessment methods, various studies have shown differing rates of adverse events from hospital to hospital. Overall, the best estimate is that approximately 1 in 10 admissions will result in an adverse event, with about half of these being preventable. Although about two-thirds of adverse events cause little or no patient harm, about one-third do—ranging from minor harm (such as a prolonged hospitalization) to permanent disability (Figure 1–2). This risk is not distributed evenly—some patients have a far higher chance of suffering a significant adverse event, and these patients may well suffer from multiple events.[15] For example, it has been estimated that the average patient in the ICU has *1.7 errors in his or her care per day in the ICU*[16] and the average hospitalized medical patient experiences *one medication error per day*[17]! Patients on multiple medications or on particularly risky medications (e.g., anticoagulants, opiates, insulin, and sedatives)[18,19] are more likely to be harmed, as are older patients (Figure 1–2).

The financial impact of medical errors and adverse events is profound. The IOM report estimated that the overall national (U.S.) costs for preventable adverse events (in the late 1990s) was between 17 billion and 29 billion dollars.[1] Including "nonpreventable" adverse events would approximately double these figures. Since these numbers come exclusively from hospital-based studies, adding in the impact of adverse events in ambulatory clinics,[20] nursing homes,[21] and other settings would drive these figures even higher.

TABLE 1–3

Advantages and disadvantages of methods used to measure errors and adverse events in healthcare

Study method	Advantages	Disadvantages
Morbidity and mortality conferences and autopsy	Can suggest contributory factors Familiar to healthcare providers	Hindsight bias Reporting bias Focused on diagnostic errors Infrequently used
Case analysis and root cause analysis	Can suggest contributory factors Structured systems approach Includes recent data from interviews	Hindsight bias Tends to focus on severe events
Malpractice claims analysis	Provides multiple perspectives (patients, providers, lawyers)	Hindsight bias Reporting bias Nonstandardized source of data
Error reporting systems	Provides multiple perspectives over time Can be a part of routine operations	Reporting bias Hindsight bias Might rely on incomplete and inaccurate data The data are divorced from the clinical context
Administrative data analysis	Uses readily available data Inexpensive	Judgments about adverse events not reliable Medical records are incomplete
Record review and chart review	Uses readily available data Commonly used	Hindsight bias
Review of electronic medical records	Inexpensive after initial investment Monitors in real time Integrates multiple data sources	Susceptible to programming and/or data entry errors Expensive to implement
Observation of patient care	Potentially accurate and precise Provides data otherwise unavailable Detects more active errors than other methods	Time consuming and expensive Difficult to train reliable observers Potential concerns about confidentiality Possible to be overwhelmed with information

Reproduced with permission from Thomas EJ, Petersen LA. Measuring errors and adverse events in health care. *J Gen Intern Med* 2003;18:61–67; Vincent C. *Patient Safety*. London: Elsevier, 2005.

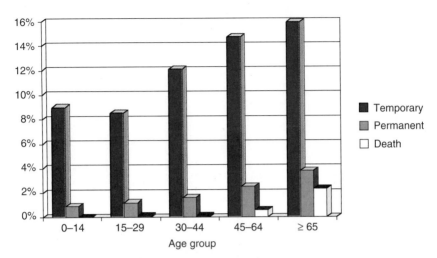

FIGURE 1–2. Proportion of patients experiencing an adverse event who suffer temporary (<1 year) disability, permanent disability, or death; by age group. Note that not only does the severity of harm go up with age, but so does the chance of an adverse event (in this Australian study it was approximately 10% per admission in younger patients, up to nearly 25% per admission in patients over 65). (Reproduced with permission from Weingart SN, Wilson RM, Gibberd RW, et al. Epidemiology of medical error. BMJ 2000;320:774-777; Wilson RM, Runciman WB, Gibberd RW, et al. The quality in Australian health care study. *Med J Aust* 1995;163:458-471.)

When viewed this way, it becomes difficult to argue that we cannot afford to fix the problem of medical errors. But—particularly in fee-for-service payment systems (like most of the United States)—part of the problem is that both providers and institutions are generally compensated (often quite handsomely) for unsafe care, providing little financial incentive to make the requisite investments in safer systems. Even in countries and organizational structures that *do* lose money from errors and harm (e.g., capitated systems such as Kaiser Permanente or the Veteran's Affairs system in the United States, or the United Kingdom's National Health Service), doing the accounting to determine the "return on investment" from spending on safety is tricky.

All of that said, one should not get too distracted by the numbers and dollars. The largest impact of medical errors and adverse events is on patients and their loved ones, and the toll is best measured in anxiety, harm, and deaths. Moreover, in so many cases, providers are "second victims" of unsafe systems that let them down when they most needed the support.[22] For all of these reasons, the moral and ethical case for patient safety remains the most powerful motivator of all.

KEY POINTS

- The modern patient safety movement began with the publication of the Institute of Medicine's report on medical errors, *To Err is Human: Building a Safer Health System,* in late 1999.
- Adverse events are injuries resulting from medical care, as opposed to adverse outcomes arising from underlying disease. Not all adverse events are preventable—those that are usually involve errors. However, in some cases preventability will involve the adoption of system changes that reduce the likelihood of the adverse events in question.
- Errors are acts of commission (doing something wrong) or omission (failing to do the right thing) leading to an undesirable outcome or significant potential for such an outcome.
- Measuring errors is very tricky. Most systems depend on voluntary reports by providers (incident reports), which only detect a small fraction of errors. Other methods, such as trigger tools or patient safety indicators from administrative datasets, may be overly sensitive and thus should be augmented by detailed chart review.
- From a variety of studies, about 1 in 10 hospital admissions lead to an adverse event, and about half of these are preventable. About one in three adverse events causes true patient harm.

REFERENCES

1. Kohn L, Corrigan J, Donaldson M, eds. *To Err is Human: Building a Safer Health System.* Washington, DC: Committee on Quality of Health Care in America, Institute of Medicine: National Academy Press, 2000.
2. Brennan TA, Leape LL, Laird NM, et al. Incidence of adverse events and negligence in hospitalized patients. Results of the Harvard Medical Practice Study I. *N Engl J Med* 1991;324:370–376.
3. Leape LL, Brennan TA, Laird N, et al. The nature of adverse events and negligence in hospitalized patients. Results of the Harvard Medical Practice Study II. *N Engl J Med* 1991;324:377–384.

4. Thomas EJ, Studdert DM, Burstin HR, et al. Incidence and types of adverse events and negligent care in Utah and Colorado. *Med Care* 2000;38:261–271.
5. Available at: http://webmm.ahrq.gov/glossary.aspx
6. Pronovost P, Needham D, Berenholtz S, et al. An intervention to decrease catheter-related bloodstream infections in the ICU. *N Engl J Med* 2006;355: 2725–2732.
7. Wild D, Bradley EH. The gap between nurses and residents in a community hospital's error reporting system. *Jt Comm J Qual Patient Saf* 2005;31: 13–20.
8. Thomas EJ, Lipsitz SR, Studdert DM, et al. The reliability of medical record review for estimating adverse event rates. *Ann Intern Med* 2002; 136:812–816.
9. Caplan RA, Posner KL, Cheney FW. Effect of outcome on physician judgments of appropriateness of care. *JAMA* 1991;265:1957–1960.
10. Classen DC, Pesotnik SL, Evans SR, et al. Computerized surveillance of adverse drug events in hospitalized patients. *JAMA* 1991;266: 2847–2851.
11. Hartis CE, Gum MO, Lederer JW Jr. Use of specific indicators to detect warfarin-related adverse events. *Am J Health Syst Pharm* 2005;62: 1683–1688.
12. Available at: http://www.qualityindicators.ahrq.gov/psi_overview.htm.
13. Thomas EJ, Petersen LA. Measuring errors and adverse events in health care. *J Gen Intern Med* 2003;18:61–67.
14. Leape LL. A systems analysis approach to medical error. *J Eval Clin Pract* 1997;3:213–222.
15. Weingart SN, Wilson RM, Gibberd RW, et al. Epidemiology of medical error. *BMJ* 2000;320:774–777.
16. Donchin Y, Gopher D, Olin M, et al. A look into the nature and causes of human errors in the intensive care unit. *Crit Care Med* 1995; 23:294–300.
17. Aspden P, Wolcott J, Bootman JL, et al., eds. *Preventing Medication Errors: Quality Chasm Series. Committee on Identifying and Preventing Medication Errors*. Washington, DC: National Academy Press, 2007.
18. Kanjanarat P, Winterstein AG, Johns TE, et al. Nature of preventable adverse drug events in hospitals: a literature review. *Am J Health Syst Pharm* 2003;60:1750–1759.
19. Bates DW, Boyle D, Vander Vliet M, et al. Relationship between medication errors and adverse drug events. *J Gen Intern Med* 1995;10: 199–205.
20. Gandhi TK, Weingart SN, Borus J, et al. Adverse drug events in ambulatory care. *N Engl J Med* 2003;348:1556–1564.

21. Gurwitz JH, Field TS, Avorn J, et al. Incidence and preventability of adverse drug events in nursing homes. *Am J Med* 2000;109:87–94.
22. Wu AW. Medical error: the second victim. *West J Med* 2000;172:358–359.

ADDITIONAL READINGS

Hilfiker D. Facing our mistakes. *N Engl J Med* 1984;310:118–122.

Rosenthal MM, Sutcliffe KM, eds. *Medical Error: What Do We Know? What Do We Do?* San Francisco, CA: Jossey-Bass, 2002.

Thomas EJ, Studdert DM, Newhouse JP, et al. Costs of medical injuries in Utah and Colorado. *Inquiry* 1999;36:255–264.

Vincent C. *Patient Safety*. London: Elsevier, 2005.

Vincent C. Understanding and responding to adverse events. *N Engl J Med* 2003;348:1051–1056.

CHAPTER TWO

Basic Principles of Patient Safety

THE MODERN APPROACH TO PATIENT SAFETY: SYSTEMS THINKING AND THE SWISS CHEESE MODEL

The traditional approach to medical errors has been to blame the provider directly delivering care to the patient, acting at what is sometimes called the "sharp end" of care: the doctor performing the transplant operation or diagnosing the patient's chest pain, the nurse hanging the intravenous medication, or the pharmacist preparing the chemotherapy. Over the last decade, we have recognized that this approach overlooks the fact that most errors are committed by hardworking, well-trained individuals, and such errors are unlikely to be prevented by admonishing people to be more careful, or by shaming and suing them.

The modern patient safety movement replaces "the blame and shame game" with a new approach, known as *systems thinking*. This paradigm acknowledges the human condition—namely, that humans err—and concludes that safety depends on creating systems that anticipate errors and either prevent or catch them before they cause harm. Such an approach has been the cornerstone of safety improvements in other high-risk industries but has been ignored in medicine until recently.

British psychologist James Reason's *"Swiss cheese model"* of organizational accidents has been widely embraced as a mental model for system safety[1,2] (Figure 2–1). This model, drawn from innumerable accident investigations in fields such as commercial aviation and nuclear power, emphasizes that in complex organizations, a single sharp-end error is rarely enough to cause harm. Instead, such errors must penetrate multiple incomplete layers of protection ("layers of Swiss cheese") to cause a devastating result. Reason's model highlights the need to focus less on the (futile) goal of trying to perfect human behavior and more on aiming to shrink the holes in the Swiss cheese (sometimes referred to as *latent errors*) and create multiple overlapping layers of protection to decrease the probability that the holes will ever align and let an error slip through.

The Swiss cheese model emphasizes that analyses of medical errors need to focus on their "root causes"—not just the smoking gun, sharp-end error, but all the underlying conditions that made an error possible (or, in some situations, inevitable) (Chapter 14). A number of investigators have developed schema for categorizing the root causes of errors; the most widely used, by Charles Vincent, is shown in Table 2–1.[3,4] The schema explicitly forces the error reviewer to ask whether there should have been a checklist or read back, whether the resident was too fatigued to think clearly, or whether the young nurse was too intimidated to speak up when she suspected an error.

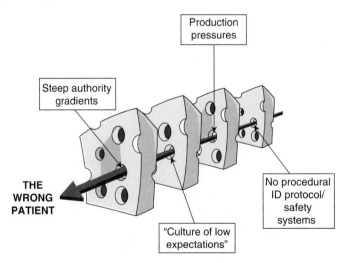

FIGURE 2–1. James Reason's Swiss cheese model of organizational accidents. The analysis is of "The Wrong Patient" case in Chapter 15. (Reproduced with permission from Reason JT. *Human Error.* New York, NY: Cambridge University Press, 1990.)

TABLE 2 – 1

Charles Vincent's framework for categorizing the root causes of errors

Framework	Contributory factors	Examples of problems that contribute to errors
Institutional	Regulatory context Medicolegal environment	Insufficient priority given by regulators to safety issues; legal pressures against open discussion, preventing the opportunity to learn from adverse events
Organization and management	Financial resources and constraints Policy standards and goals Safety culture and priorities	Lack of awareness of safety issues on the part of senior management; policies leading to inadequate staffing levels
Work environment	Staffing levels and mix of skills Patterns in workload and shifts Design, availability, and maintenance of equipment Administrative and managerial support	Heavy workloads, leading to fatigue; limited access to essential equipment; inadequate administrative support, leading to reduced time with patients
Team	Verbal communication Written communication Supervision and willingness to seek help Team leadership	Poor supervision of junior staff; poor communication among different professions; unwillingness of junior staff to seek assistance
Individual staff member	Knowledge and skills Motivation and attitude Physical and mental health	Lack of knowledge or experience; long-term fatigue and stress
Task	Availability and use of protocols Availability and accuracy of test results	Unavailability of test results or delay in obtaining them; lack of clear protocols and guidelines
Patient	Complexity and seriousness of condition Language and communication Personality and social factors	Distress; language barriers between patients and caregivers

Reproduced with permission from Vincent C. Understanding and responding to adverse events. *N Engl J Med* 2003;348:1051–1056; Vincent C, Taylor-Adams S, Stanhope N. Framework for analyzing risk and safety in clinical medicine. *BMJ* 1998;316:1154–1157.

ERRORS AT THE SHARP END: SLIPS VERSUS MISTAKES

Even though we now understand that the root cause of hundreds of thousands of errors each year lies at the "blunt end," the proximate cause is often an act committed (or neglected, or performed incorrectly) by a caregiver. While embracing the systems approach as the most useful paradigm, it would be wrong not to tackle these human errors as well. After all, even a room filled with flammable gas will not explode unless a person strikes a match.

In thinking about human errors, it is useful to differentiate between "slips" and "mistakes"; and to do this, one must appreciate the difference between *conscious* behavior and *automatic* behavior. Conscious behavior is what we do when we "pay attention" to a task, and it is especially important when we are doing something new, like learning to play the piano or program our DVD player. On the other hand, automatic behaviors are the things we do almost unconsciously—they may have required a lot of thought initially, but after a while we do them virtually "in our sleep." Humans prefer automatic behaviors because they take less energy, have predictable outcomes, and allow us to "multitask"—do other things at the same time. Some of these other tasks are also automatic behaviors, like driving a car while drinking coffee or talking on the phone, but some require conscious thought. These latter moments—when a doctor tries to write a "routine" prescription while also pondering his approach to a challenging patient—are particularly risky, both for making errors in the routine, automatic process ("slips") or in the conscious process ("mistakes").

Now that we've distinguished the two types of tasks, let's turn to slips versus mistakes. *Slips* are inadvertent, unconscious lapses in the performance of some automatic task. You absently drive to work on Sunday morning because your automatic behavior kicks in and dictates your actions. Slips occur most often when we put an activity on "autopilot" so we can manage new sensory inputs, think through a problem, or deal with emotional upset, fatigue, or stress (a pretty good description of most healthcare environments). *Mistakes*, on the other hand, result from incorrect choices. Rather than blundering into them while we are distracted, they usually result from insufficient knowledge, lack of experience or training, inadequate information (or inability to interpret available information properly), or applying the wrong set of rules or algorithms to a decision.

Although on an "errors per action" yardstick, conscious behaviors are more prone to mistakes than automatic behaviors are prone to slips;

slips probably represent the greater overall threat to patient safety because so much of what healthcare providers do is automatic. Doctors and nurses are most likely to slip while doing something they have done correctly a thousand times—asking patients if they are allergic to any medications before writing a prescription, remembering to verify a patient's identity before sending them off to a procedure, or loading a syringe with heparin (and not insulin) before flushing an IV line (the latter case will be described in Chapter 4).

The complexity of healthcare work adds to the risks. Like pilots, soldiers, and others trained to work in high-risk occupations, doctors and nurses are programmed to do many specific tasks, under pressure, with a high degree of accuracy. But unlike most other professions, medical jobs typically combine three very different types of tasks: lots of conscious behaviors (complex decisions, judgment calls), lots of "customer" interactions, and innumerable automatic behaviors. Physician training, in particular, has traditionally emphasized the decision making, highly cognitive aspects, focused a bit on the human interactions, and completely ignored the importance, and risky nature, of automatic behaviors.

With all of this in mind, how then should we respond to the inevitability of slips? Our typical response would be to reprimand (if not fire) a nurse for giving the wrong medication, and admonish her to "look more carefully next time!" Even if the nurse did, she is just as likely to commit a different error while automatically carrying out a different task in a different setting. As James Reason reminds us, "Errors are largely unintentional. It is very difficult for management to control what people did not intend to do in the first place."[2] And it is not just managers whose instinct is to blame the provider at the sharp end—we providers blame ourselves! When we make a slip—a stupid error in something that we usually do perfectly "in our sleep"—we feel embarrassed. We chastise ourselves harder than any supervisor could, and swear we'll never make a careless mistake like that again. Realistically, though, such promises are almost impossible to keep.

Whatever the strategy employed to prevent slips (and they will be discussed throughout the book), a clear lesson is that boring, repetitive tasks can be dangerous and are often performed better by machines. In medicine, these tasks include monitoring a patient's oxygen level during a long surgery, suturing large wounds, holding surgical retractors steady for a long time, and scanning mountains of data for significant patterns. Anesthesiologist Alan Merry and legal scholar and novelist Alexander McCall Smith observe, people have no need to apologize for their failure to achieve machine-like standards in those activities for which machines are better suited. They are good at other things—original thought, for one, empathy and compassion for another. . . It is true that people are distractible—but in fact this provides a major survival advantage for them. A machine (unless expressly designed to detect such an event) will continue with its repetitive task while the house burns down around it, whereas most humans will notice that something unexpected is going on and will change their activity. . .[5]

GENERAL PRINCIPLES OF PATIENT SAFETY IMPROVEMENT STRATEGIES

Drawing on these mental models, the modern patient safety field emphasizes the need to shore up systems to prevent or catch errors rather than to create "goof-proof" individual providers. For example, errors in routine behaviors ("slips") can best be prevented by *building in redundancies and cross checks*, in the form of checklists, read backs ("let me read your order back to you"), and other standardized safety procedures (e.g., signing the surgical site prior to an operation, asking patients their name before medication administration). It also emphasizes the need for *standardization and simplification*. For example, if the process of taking a patient to the MRI scanner is standardized, it is far more likely that the correct safety procedures can be "baked in" and deviations from them noticed and rectified. Recently, there has been increased emphasis on decreasing errors at the person-machine interface through the use of *forcing functions*—engineering solutions that decrease the probability of human error. The classic example outside medicine was the changes made to automobile braking systems that rendered it impossible to place a car in reverse when the driver's foot is off the brake. In healthcare, forcing functions include changing the gas nozzles and connectors so that anesthesiologists cannot mistakenly hook up the wrong gas to a patient. Given the ever-increasing complexity of modern medicine, building in such forcing functions (in intravenous pumps, cardiac defibrillators, mechanical ventilators, and computerized order entry systems) will be crucial to safety (Chapter 7).

In addition to systems enhancements, there has been a growing recognition of the importance of improving communication and teamwork. Commercial pilots all participate in "crew resource management" courses in which they train for emergencies with other crew, learning to create flatter hierarchies to encourage open communication, communicate clearly using standard language, and utilize checklists, debriefings, and other systemic approaches. Although the evidence that such interventions will improve patient safety is preliminary,[6] there is considerable enthusiasm about them in safety circles. The term "culture of safety" is used as shorthand for an environment in which teamwork, clear communication, and openness about errors (both to other healthcare professionals and to patients) are operative (Chapter 15).

Another key patient safety principle is to learn from one's mistakes. This may take multiple forms. Safe systems have a culture in which errors are openly discussed, often in morbidity and mortality (M&M) conferences. There is a new push to make sure that such discussions include members of the appropriate disciplines (nursing, hospital administration, not just physicians), point out errors rather than gloss over them in the name of avoiding a punitive atmosphere, and emphasize systems thinking and solutions.[7] In addition to the open discussion at conferences, safe organizations build in mechanisms to hear about errors from frontline staff, often via incident reporting systems (Chapter 1) or unit-based safety teams,[8] and to perform detailed ("root cause") analyses of major errors ("sentinel events") in an effort to define all the "layers of Swiss cheese" that need attention (Chapter 14).

Finally, there is increasing appreciation of the importance of a well-trained, well-staffed, and well-rested workforce in delivering safe care. There is now evidence linking low nurse-to-patient ratios, long resident work hours, and lack of board certification to poor patient outcomes.[9–13] Such research is catalyzing a more holistic view of patient safety, recognizing that the implementation of "safer systems" will not create safe patient care if the providers are overextended, poorly trained, or under supervised.

This long list of potential approaches to improving safety (each of which will be discussed in greater detail later in the book) highlights one of the great challenges in the field: in the absence of comparative evidence, and in light of the high cost of some of the interventions (e.g., improved staffing, computerized order entry, teamwork training), even institutions committed to safety can become bewildered as they consider which approach to emphasize.[14] Institutions quite naturally focus on the practices that are measured, publicly reported, and compensated. As the next chapter will show, such a prioritization scheme will tend to elevate quality improvement strategies over those focused on patient safety, because the results of the former are easier to measure. This raises the importance of regulatory approaches (such as standards set by the Joint Commission) (Chapter 20). Thankfully, many of the approaches to improving quality, such as computerization and standardization, will also yield safety benefits. On the other hand, because improving culture is both difficult and hard to measure, publicly report, and regulate, it may end up being shuffled to the bottom of the deck, notwithstanding its importance to patient safety. Pronovost, Miller, and I have suggested a measurement scheme for patient safety that takes these considerations into account, and includes elements of safety culture[15] (Table 2–2).

KEY POINTS

- The modern approach to patient safety hinges on "systems thinking"— a recognition that most errors are made by competent, careful, and caring providers, and preventing these errors often involves embedding the providers in a system that anticipates glitches and catches them before they do harm.

TABLE 2–2

A proposed method for measuring progress in patient safety

Measures that can be feasibly captured as rates

1. How often are patients harmed? (e.g., rates of healthcare-acquired infections, postoperative venous thromboembolism, or medication errors)
2. How often do clinicians provide appropriate interventions? (e.g., measures of processes that have been strongly linked to safety outcomes: higher nurse-to-patient ratios, pharmacist presence on hospital units, functioning computerized provider order entry)

Measures that generally cannot be presented as rates

1. Have clinicians learned from mistakes? (evidence that incident reports or root cause analyses led to meaningful changes, such as new policies or procedures)
2. How successful are clinicians and healthcare systems in creating a culture of safety? (has the system administered a validated safety culture survey to the staff, and demonstrated improvement on it?)

Reproduced with permission from Pronovost PJ, Miller MR, Wachter RM. Tracking progress in patient safety: an elusive target. *JAMA* 2006;296: 696–699.

- James Reason's "Swiss cheese model" is the dominant paradigm for understanding the relationship between active ("sharp end") errors and latent ("blunt end") errors; it is important to resist the temptation to focus solely on the former and neglect the latter.

- A variety of strategies should be employed to create safer systems, including simplification, standardization, using redundancies, improving teamwork and communication, and learning from past mistakes.

REFERENCES

1. Reason JT. *Human Error*. New York, NY: Cambridge University Press, 1990.
2. Reason JT. *Managing the Risks of Organizational Accidents*. Aldershot, Hampshire, England: Ashgate, 1997.
3. Vincent C. Understanding and responding to adverse events. *N Engl J Med* 2003;348:1051–1056.
4. Vincent C, Taylor-Adams S, Stanhope N. Framework for analyzing risk and safety in clinical medicine. *BMJ* 1998;316:1154–1157.
5. Merry A, Smith AM. *Errors, Medicine, and the Law*. Cambridge, England: Cambridge University Press, 2001.
6. Salas E, Wilson KA, Burke CS, et al. Does crew resource management training work? An update, an extension, and some critical needs. *Hum Factors* 2006;48:392–412.
7. Pierluissi E, Fischer MA, Campbell AR, et al. Discussion of medical errors in morbidity and mortality conferences. *JAMA* 2003;290: 2838–2842.
8. Pronovost P, Weast B, Rosenstein B. Implementing and validating a comprehensive unit-based safety program. *J Patient Saf* 2005;1:33–40.
9. Aiken LH, Clarke SP, Sloane DM, et al. Hospital nurse staffing and patient mortality, nurse burnout, and job dissatisfaction. *JAMA* 2002;288: 1987–1993.
10. Landrigan CP, Rothschild JM, Cronin JW, et al. Effect of reducing interns' work hours on serious medical errors in intensive care units. *N Engl J Med* 2004;351:1838–1848.
11. Brennan TA, Horwitz RI, Duffy FD, et al. The role of physician specialty board certification status in the quality movement. *JAMA* 2004;292: 1038–1043.

12. Hugonnet S, Chevrolet JC, Pittet D. The effect of workload on infection risk in critically ill patients. *Crit Care Med* 2007;35:76–81.
13. Ong M, Bostrom A, Vidyarthi A, et al. House staff team workload and organization effects on patient outcomes in an academic general internal medicine inpatient service. *Arch Intern Med* 2007;167:47–52.
14. Wachter RM. The end of the beginning: patient safety five years after "To Err is Human." *Health Aff (Millwood)* 2004;(Suppl W4):534–545.
15. Pronovost PJ, Miller MR, Wachter RM. Tracking progress in patient safety: an elusive target. *JAMA* 2006;296:696–699.

ADDITIONAL READINGS

Gaba DM. Structural and organizational issues in patient safety: a comparison of health care to other high-hazard industries. *Calif Manage Rev* 2000; 43:1–20.

Helmreich RL. On error management: lessons from aviation. *BMJ* 2000; 320:781–785.

Leape LL. Error in medicine. *JAMA* 1994;272:1851–1857.

Longo DR, Hewett JE, Ge B, et al. The long road to patient safety: a status report on patient safety systems. *JAMA* 2005;294:2858–2865.

Reason J. Beyond the organizational accident: the need for "error wisdom" on the frontline. *Qual Saf Health Care* 2004;13(Suppl 2):ii28–ii33.

Wachter RM, Shojania KG. *Internal Bleeding: The Truth Behind America's Terrifying Epidemic of Medical Mistakes*. New York, NY: Rugged Land, 2004.

CHAPTER THREE

Safety Versus Quality

WHAT IS QUALITY?

Quality of care has been defined by the Institute of Medicine (IOM) as "the degree to which health services for individuals and populations increase the likelihood of desired health outcomes and are consistent with current professional knowledge." In its influential 2001 report, *Crossing the Quality Chasm*, the IOM advanced six aims for a quality healthcare system (Table 3–1): patient safety, patient-centeredness, effectiveness, efficiency, timeliness, and equity.[1] Note that safety is depicted as one of the six components, in essence making it a subset of quality. Note also that, though many clinicians tend to think of quality as being synonymous with the delivery of evidence-based care, the IOM's definition is much broader and includes matters that are of particular importance to patients (patient-centeredness and timeliness) and to society (equity).

Although the IOM makes clear that quality is more than the provision of care supported by science, evidence-based medicine does provide the foundation for much of quality measurement and improvement. For many decades, promoted by a lack of clinical evidence and the apprenticeship model of medical training, the idiosyncratic practice style of a senior clinician or a prestigious medical center determined the standard of care (a tradition now sometimes termed "eminence-based medicine," with more than a hint of derision). Without discounting the value of experience and mature clinical judgment, the modern paradigm for identifying optimal practice has changed, driven by the explosion in clinical research over the past two generations (the number of randomized clinical trials has grown from less than 500 per year in 1970 to 15,000 per year in 2006). This research has helped define "best practices" in many areas of

TABLE 3–1
The IOM's six aims for a quality healthcare system
• Healthcare must be safe
• Healthcare must be effective
• Healthcare must be patient-centered
• Healthcare must be timely
• Healthcare must be efficient
• Healthcare must be equitable

Reproduced with permission from Committee on Quality of Health Care in America, Institute of Medicine. *Crossing the Quality Chasm: A New Health System for the 21st Century.* Washington, DC: National Academy Press, 2001.

medicine, from preventive strategies for a 64-year-old woman with diabetes to the treatment of the patient with acute myocardial infarction and cardiogenic shock.

The health services researcher Avedis Donabedian provided a ground-breaking taxonomy for measuring the quality of care. "Donabedian's Triad" divides quality measures into *structure* (how is care organized), *process* (what was done), and *outcomes* (what happened to the patient).[2] Each element of the Triad has important advantages and disadvantages[3] (Table 3–2). In recent years, as clinical research has established the link between certain processes and improved outcomes, the trend has been toward the use of process measurement as proxies for quality. Examples include measuring the glycosylated hemoglobin at appropriate intervals in outpatients with diabetes or whether hospitalized patients with pneumonia received influenza and pneumococcal vaccination. However, when processes-outcome links are less well established and the science of case-mix adjustment is suitably advanced (e.g., cardiac bypass surgery), outcome measurement is often used. The latter caveat is crucial: if case-mix adjustment is not done well, the surgeon or hospital who accepts (or is referred) the sickest patients will appear to be worse than the lesser surgeon or institution that only takes easy cases. Finally, when the processes are quite complex and the science of case-mix adjustment is immature, structural measures are used as proxies for quality (assuming that good research has linked such structural elements to overall quality). Examples here include the presence of intensivists in critical care units, a dedicated stroke service, and computerized provider order entry (CPOE).

TABLE 3–2

Advantages and disadvantages of using structure, process, and outcome (the "Donabedian Triad") to measure the quality of care

Measure	Simple definition	Advantages	Disadvantages
Structure	How was care organized?	May be highly relevant in a complex health system	May fail to capture the quality of care by individual physicians Difficult to determine the "gold standard"
Process	What was done?	More easily measured and acted upon than outcomes May not require case-mix adjustment No time lag—can be measured when care is provided May directly reflect quality (if carefully chosen)	A proxy for outcomes All may not agree on "gold standard" processes May promote "cookbook" medicine, especially if physicians and health systems try to "game" their performance
Outcome	What happened to the patient?	What we really care about	May take years to occur May not reflect quality of care Requires case-mix and other adjustment to prevent "apples-to-oranges" comparisons

Reproduced with permission from Shojania KG, Showstack J, Wachter RM. Assessing hospital quality: a review for clinicians. *Eff Clin Pract* 2001;4:82–90.

THE EPIDEMIOLOGY OF QUALITY PROBLEMS

Wennberg's pioneering studies demonstrating large and clinically inde-fensible variations in care from one city to another for the same problem or procedure were the first to show widespread deviations from best prac-tices.[4] Other studies have demonstrated large variations in the quality of care for patients based on race, income, and gender ("healthcare dispari-ties").[5] Together, these studies hint at a fundamental flaw in modern med-ical practice; namely, to create such profound variations in the frequency of even common processes and procedures, much of our care must not be consistent with evidence.

More recently, researchers have more directly measured the fre-quency with which doctors and healthcare organizations provide care that comports with best evidence. McGlynn and colleagues studied more than 400 evidence-based measures of quality, and found that practice was consistent with the evidence only 54% of the time.[6] Adherence to evidence-based processes generally correlates with ultimate clinical outcomes,[7] although some recent studies have found a weaker relationship than one would anticipate.[8, 9] Nevertheless, these large differences between best and actual practice have caused patients, providers, and policymakers to search for methods to drive and support quality improvement (QI) activities.

CATALYSTS FOR QUALITY IMPROVEMENT

The problems described above have exposed several impediments to the reliable delivery of high quality care, including: the lack of information regarding provider or institutional performance, the weakness of incen-tives for QI, the difficulty for practicing physicians to stay abreast of evi-dence-based medicine, and the absence of system support (such as information technology) for quality. Each will need to be addressed in order to make substantial gains in the quality of care.

The first step in QI begins with *quality measurement*. A decade ago, there were only a handful of generally accepted quality measures, such as whether patients with acute myocardial infarction received aspirin or beta-blockers. More recently, literally scores of such measures have been promul-gated by a variety of organizations, including payers (such as the Centers for Medicare & Medicaid Services [CMS]), accreditors and regulators (such as the Joint Commission), and medical societies (Table 3–3). These measures have identified many opportunities for individual physicians, practices, and hospitals to improve.

Given the enormous amount of new literature each year, no individual physician can possibly remain abreast of all the evidence-based advances in his or her field. *Practice guidelines*, such as those for the care of community-acquired pneumonia or for prophylaxis for deep venous

---

TABLE 3–3

Examples of publicly reported quality measures

Acute myocardial infarction measures

Aspirin at arrival
Aspirin at discharge
ACE inhibitor or ARB for LVS dysfunction
Beta-blocker at arrival
Beta-blocker at discharge
Thrombolytic agent received within 30 min of hospital arrival
Percutaneous coronary intervention (PCI) received within 120 min of hospital arrival
Smoking cessation advice/counseling

Heart failure measures

Evaluation of LVS function
ACE inhibitor or ARB for LVS dysfunction
Discharge instructions
Smoking cessation advice/counseling

Pneumonia measures

Oxygenation assessment
Initial antibiotic timing
Pneumococcal vaccination
Influenza vaccination
Blood culture performed in the ED prior to initial antibiotic received in hospital
Appropriate initial antibiotic selection
Smoking cessation advice/counseling

Surgical care improvement/surgical infection prevention measures

Prophylactic antibiotic received within 1 h of surgical incision
Prophylactic antibiotics discontinued within 24 h after surgery end time

---

Abbreviations: ACE, angiotensin-converting enzyme; ARB, angiotensin-receptor blocker; LVS, left ventricular systolic.
Reproduced with permission from the Hospital Quality Alliance and the CMS. Available at: http://www.hospitalcompare.hhs.gov/Hospital/Static/Data-Professionals.asp?dest= NAV|Home|DataDetails|ProfessionalInfo#measureset.

thrombosis, aim to synthesize evidence-based best practices into sets of summary recommendations. Although some providers deride guidelines as "cookbook medicine," there is increasing agreement that standardizing best practices is ethically and clinically appropriate; in fact, "high reliability organizations" "hard wire" such practices whenever possible. The major challenges for guideline developers are the need to keep guidelines updated as new knowledge accumulates[10] and the difficulties in remaining relevant to the care of patients with multiple, potentially overlapping illnesses.[11] *Clinical pathways* are similar to guidelines, but attempt to articulate a series of steps, usually temporal (on day one, do the following; on day two ...). Therefore, they are generally more useful for stereotypical processes such as the postoperative management of patients after cardiac bypass surgery or hip replacement.

THE CHANGING QUALITY LANDSCAPE

Although one could argue that professionalism should be sufficient incentive to provide high quality care, our recent recognition that the unwavering provision of such care often depends on a system organized to reliably translate research into practice means that it will take significant investments (i.e., in physician education, hiring case managers or clinical pharmacists, building information systems, and developing guidelines) to deliver optimal care. The traditional payment system, which compensates physicians and hospitals equally whether quality is superb or appalling, provides no incentive to make the requisite investments.

This is changing rapidly, with a blizzard of recent initiatives to support and catalyze QI activities. Virtually all involve several steps: defining reasonable quality measures (evidence-based measures that capture appropriate structures, processes, or outcomes), measuring the performance of providers or systems, and using these results to promote change. Although each of these steps comes with challenges, it is the final one that creates the greatest degree of uncertainty and has been the subject of the greatest amount of experimentation.

Although one might hope that simply feeding back individual providers' performance to themselves will generate meaningful improvement, experience has shown that this strategy leads to only modest change. Increasingly, a more aggressive strategy of *transparency* (disseminating the results of quality measures to key stakeholders) is becoming the norm. With simple transparency, the hope is that providers will find the public dissemination of their quality gaps to be sufficiently concerning to motivate improvement. Further, many believe that patients (or their proxies, such as third party payers) will begin to use such data to make choices about where patients receive care. To date, there is little evidence that patients are using such data to make purchasing decisions. Nevertheless, studies have shown impressive improvements in some publicly reported quality measures, supporting the premise that transparency itself may generate change.[12]

The newest strategy is to tie payments for service to quality performance (*Pay for Performance*, or "P4P").[13] Although P4P is conceptually attractive, it also raises a host of concerns, including over whether quality data are accurate, whether payments should go to best performers or those with the greatest improvements, whether existing measures adequately measure quality in patients with complex, multiorgan disease, and whether P4P will create undue focus on measurable practices and relative inattention to other important process that are not being compensated.[14, 15] At this writing, a number of experiments are testing the impact of P4P in a variety of settings. Early evidence from these experiments indicates that P4P may create somewhat more change than that generated by transparency alone; the jury is still out on whether this marginal benefit (if it in fact exists) is enough to overcome the concerns cited above.[16,17]

QUALITY IMPROVEMENT STRATEGIES

Whether the motivation is ethics, embarrassment, or economics, the next question is how to actually improve the quality of care. There is no simple answer. In general, most institutions and physicians that have been successful in this work use a variation of a "Plan-Do-Study-Act" (PDSA) cycle (Figure 3–1), recognizing that QI activities must be carefully planned and implemented, that their impact needs to be measured, and that the results of these activities need to be fed back into the system in a continuously iterative process of improvement.

In addition to the PDSA cycle, several other tactics are useful. For QI practices that require predictable repetition, efforts to "hard wire" the practice or use alternative providers who focus on the activity are often beneficial. For example, the strategy most likely to increase the rate of pneumococcal vaccination of hospitalized patients with pneumonia is to embed it in a standard order set (either paper-based or computerized). Having a nurse remove the patient's shoes before the doctor enters the room can increase rates of diabetic foot examinations in outpatient practice.

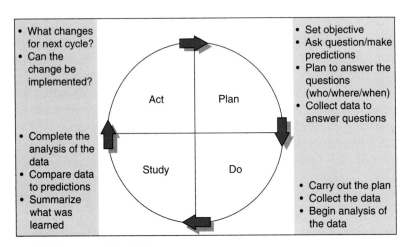

- What changes for next cycle?
- Can the change be implemented?

- Complete the analysis of the data
- Compare data to predictions
- Summarize what was learned

Act

Plan

Study

Do

- Set objective
- Ask question/make predictions
- Plan to answer the questions (who/where/when)
- Collect data to answer questions

- Carry out the plan
- Collect the data
- Begin analysis of the data

FIGURE 3–1. The PDSA cycle.

In some areas, though, QI involves much more complex and interdependent activities. In these circumstances, bringing teams together to examine their practices and participate in a PDSA cycle is the most likely path to success. For example, a group of cardiac surgeons in the northeastern United States participated in a multicenter QI project in which they observed each other's practices, agreed upon best practices, and scrutinized each other's outcomes and suggested improvement strategies. The result: a 24% reduction in cardiac surgery mortality.[18]

COMMONALITIES AND DIFFERENCES BETWEEN QUALITY AND SAFETY

Although patient safety is a subset of the larger issue of quality of care, it is important to appreciate the sometimes blurred differences between the two areas, particularly regarding measuring performance and changing practices and systems.

Mr. S, a 74-year-old man, is admitted to the hospital with severe substernal chest pain. In the emergency department (ED), his electrocardiogram (ECG) shows the ST elevation typical of a significant myocardial infarction. In this hospital, ST-elevation myocardial infarctions are managed with emergent balloon angioplasty, and there is strong evidence linking "door-to-balloon

*times" to ultimate outcome. There is a delay in reaching the cardi-
ologist on call; when he finally arrives an hour later, the cardiac
catheterization lab is not prepared for the procedure, leading to
another delay. The cardiologist, Dr. G, orders a dose of metoprolol, a beta-blocker. Dr. G's handwriting is difficult to read, but the
pharmacist is reluctant to page the doctor, who is known for his
"difficult personality." So the pharmacist takes his best guess at
the prescription and dispenses a dose of metformin, a medicine
for diabetes. Ultimately, the mistake is recognized and the correct
medicine is administered as the patient is being wheeled up for his
angioplasty. The door-to-balloon time is 150 minutes, well above
the goal of 90 minutes or less. The patient survives, but is left
with a moderate amount of heart damage (ejection fraction 35%,
normal 55–70%) and mildly symptomatic heart failure.*

This case illustrates both quality and safety problems. The administration of the wrong medicine (metformin instead of metoprolol) is clearly an
error. Future approaches to preventing such errors would likely include
computerization, standardization, and changes in culture that would
ensure that the pharmacist would promptly call the physician to clarify an
ambiguous order. But the prolonged door-to-balloon time also represents a
quality problem, a failure in the process of care. There were no overt
errors in this process, it just took far longer than it should have because of
lack of coordination, planning, and training. The combined result of both
kinds of problems was a poor outcome: limited functional status and
diminished ejection fraction.

Differentiating the quality and safety problems is important as we
consider their causes and how best to prevent them. Let's assume that the
patient's insurer was interested in measuring the quality and safety of
care in this hospital. It would be relatively easy to implement a transparent,
auditable process to measure the door-to-balloon time. Ditto for
whether the patient received aspirin, a beta-blocker, or a flu shot at discharge. Turning to outcomes, it would be straightforward to figure out
whether Mr. S and similar patients were alive or dead at the time of discharge (though remember that we'd need some pretty sophisticated case-
mix adjustment to be sure that our outcome assessment wasn't unfairly
disadvantaging the hospital or doctors that attract sicker patients). Public
reporting of door-to-balloon times, perhaps accompanied by higher reim-
bursement for better performance (via P4P), would likely lead to
improved performance.

But how could this insurer learn of Mr. S's medication error? It is difficult to imagine a transparent, auditable system that does not depend on the nurse, pharmacist, or physician's self-report to capture the error. Moreover, a strategy of public reporting (or P4P) for medication errors might well leave providers reluctant to report them, causing the system to be unaware that such errors were occurring and ill prepared to generate the shared knowledge—as well as the money and will—to fix them.

The process of fixing both problems (door-to-balloon times and medication errors) might be relatively similar, in that both are likely to require changes in core processes (all patients with chest pain will receive ECGs in the first 5 minutes of arriving in the ED; all prescriptions will include medication name, dose, and indication), thoughtful implementation of technology (perhaps an automatic ECG reader for the chest pain protocol; CPOE for the medication error), and changes in culture (simulation training to improve door-to-balloon time performance; teamwork training to improve physician-pharmacist communication and dampen down hierarchies for the medication error).

The bottom line is that patients have a right to expect care that is both high quality and safe. The IOM report on medical errors, *To Err is Human*, helped catalyze a national push to improve safety, and has led to important changes in culture, training, regulation, and technology.[19] However, because measuring safety tends to depend largely on providers' self-report, the twin strategies of transparency and differential payment have more relevance to efforts to improve quality than safety.[20] Happily, the two endeavors have enough commonalities (the need for improved information systems, standardization, and simplification, use of multidisciplinary teams, and improvement cycles) that QI initiatives will also result in better safety. Other cornerstones of patient safety, such as the creation of a safety culture (Chapter 15), may be largely independent of QI efforts and will require a distinct focus.

KEY POINTS

- Safety is usually considered to be a subset of quality, but it is more difficult to measure, in part because identification of incidents often depends on self-reports by caregivers.
- There is tremendous activity in the healthcare marketplace promoting transparency in quality measurement and possible differential payment for better performance ("P4P").

- Quality measurement is usually organized around "Donebedian's Triad": structure, process, or outcomes, with each type of measure having advantages and disadvantages when compared with the others.

REFERENCES

1. Committee on Quality of Health Care in America, Institute of Medicine. *Crossing the Quality Chasm: A New Health System for the 21st Century.* Washington, DC: National Academy Press, 2001.
2. Donabedian A. The quality of care. How can it be assessed? *JAMA* 1988;260:1743–1748.
3. Shojania KG, Showstack J, Wachter RM. Assessing hospital quality: a review for clinicians. *Eff Clin Pract* 2001;4:82–90.
4. Wennberg JE, Freeman JL, Culp WJ. Are hospital services rationed in New Haven or over-utilised in Boston? *Lancet* 1987;1:1185–1189.
5. Committee on Understanding and Eliminating Racial and Ethnic Disparities in Health Care, 2003, Institute of Medicine. *Unequal Treatment: Confronting Racial and Ethnic Disparities in Health Care.* Washington, DC: National Academy Press, 2003.
6. McGlynn EA, Asch SM, Adams J, et al. The quality of health care delivered to adults in the United States. *N Engl J Med* 2003;348:2635–2645.
7. Higashi T, Shekelle PG, Adams JL, et al. Quality of care is associated with survival in vulnerable older patients. *Ann Intern Med* 2005;143:274–281.
8. Bradley EH, Herrin J, Elbel B, et al. Hospital quality for acute myocardial infarction: correlation among process measures and relationship with short-term mortality. *JAMA* 2006;296:72–78.
9. Fonarow GC, Abraham WT, Albert NM, et al. Association between performance measures and clinical outcomes for patients hospitalized with heart failure. *JAMA* 2007;297:61–70.
10. Shekelle PG, Ortiz E, Rhodes S, et al. Validity of the Agency for Healthcare Research and Quality clinical practice guidelines: how quickly do guidelines become outdated? *JAMA* 2001;286:1461–1467.
11. Boyd CM, Darer J, Boult C, et al. Clinical practice guidelines and quality of care for older patients with multiple comorbid diseases: implications for pay for performance. *JAMA* 2005;294:716–724.
12. Williams SC, Schmaltz SP, Morton DJ, et al. Quality of care in U.S. hospitals as reflected by standardized measures, 2002–2004. *N Engl J Med* 2005;353:255–264.
13. Fisher ES. Paying for performance—risks and recommendations. *N Engl J Med* 2006;355:1845–1847.
14. Rosenthal MB, Frank RG, Li Z, et al. Early experience with pay-for-performance: from concept to practice. *JAMA* 2005;294:1788–1793.

15. Wachter RM. Expected and unanticipated consequences of the quality and information technology revolutions. *JAMA* 2006;295:2780–2783.

16. Lindenauer PK, Remus D, Roman S, et al. Public reporting and pay for performance in hospital quality improvement. *N Engl J Med* 2007; 356:486–496.

17. Glickman SW, Ou F, DeLong ER, et al. Pay for performance, quality of care, and outcomes in acute myocardial infarction. *JAMA* 2007;297: 2373–2380.

18 O'Connor GT, Plume SK, Olmstead EM, et al. A regional intervention to improve the hospital mortality associated with coronary artery bypass graft surgery. The Northern New England Cardiovascular Disease Study Group. *JAMA* 1996;275:841–846.

19. Kohn LT, Corrigan JM, Donaldson MS, eds. *To Err is Human: Building a Safer Health System*. Washington, DC: National Academy Press, 2000.

20. Pronovost PJ, Miller MR, Wachter RM. Tracking progress in patient safety: an elusive target. *JAMA* 2006;296:696–699.

ADDITIONAL READINGS

Brennan TA, Gawande A, Thomas E, et al. Accidental deaths, saved lives, and improved quality. *N Engl J Med* 2005;353:1405–1409.

Fisher ES, Wennberg DE, Stukel TA, et al. The implications of regional variations in Medicare spending. Part 1: the content, quality, and accessibility of care. *Ann Intern Med* 2003;138:273–287.

Fisher ES, Wennberg DE, Stukel TA, et al. The implications of regional variations in Medicare spending. Part 2: health outcomes and satisfaction with care. *Ann Intern Med* 2003;138:288–298.

Horn SD. Performance measures and clinical outcomes. *JAMA* 2006;296: 2731–2732.

Millenson ML. *Demanding Medical Excellence. Doctors and Accountability in the Information Age*. Chicago, IL: University of Chicago Press, 1997.

Pronovost PJ, Nolan T, Zeger S, et al. How can clinicians measure safety and quality in acute care? *Lancet* 2004;363:1061–1067.

Types of Medical Errors

CHAPTER FOUR

Medication Errors

SOME BASIC CONCEPTS, TERMS, AND EPIDEMIOLOGY

*I*n *June 1995, a middle-aged man named Ramon Vasquez went to see his physician in Odessa, Texas to investigate his chest pain. His physician, suspecting angina, prescribed a medication. The actual prescription is reproduced in Figure 4–1.*

Here's a quiz. Do you think the highlighted portion of the prescription is for

- **a.** Plendil, a calcium channel blocker sometimes used to treat angina
- **b.** Isordil, a long-acting nitrate also used to treat angina
- **c.** Zestril, an angiotensin-converting enzyme inhibitor used to treat high blood pressure and heart failure

So what did you think? I once asked an audience of hospitalists to interpret this prescription. Half said it was Plendil, one-third Isordil, and the rest Zestril.

The physician actually intended to prescribe 120 tablets of Isordil, at its typical dose of 20 milligrams (mg) by mouth (po) every (Q) six hours. Ramon Vasquez's pharmacist read the prescription as Plendil, and instructed the patient to take a 20 milligram pill every six hours. Unfortunately, the usual starting dose of Plendil is 10 mg/day, making this an eightfold overdose. A day later, Mr. Vasquez was critically ill from low blood pressure and heart failure. He died within the week.

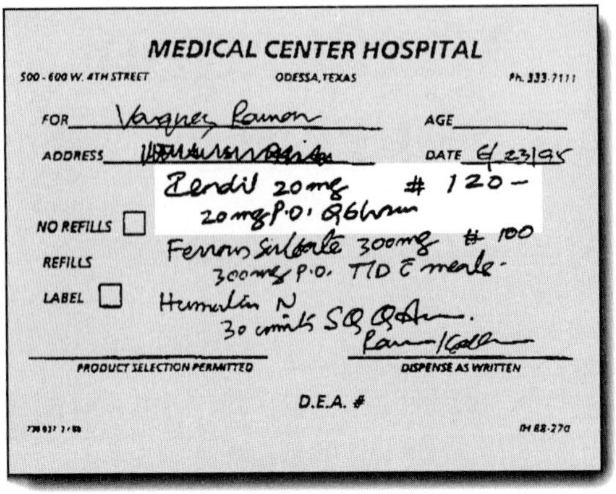
MEDICAL CENTER HOSPITAL

500-600 W. 4TH STREET ODESSA, TEXAS Ph. 333-7111

FOR Vasquez Ramon AGE

ADDRESS DATE 6/23/95

NO REFILLS

REFILLS

LABEL

Zendil 20 mg # 120 —
20 mg P.O. Q6 hours

Ferrous Sulfate 300mg # 100
300mg P.O. TID c̄ meals.

Humulin N
30 units SQ Q Am.

PRODUCT SELECTION PERMITTED

DISPENSE AS WRITTEN

D.E.A. #

FIGURE 4–1. Ramon Vasquez's prescription.

The modern pharmaceutical armamentarium represents one of healthcare's great advances. There are now highly effective agents to treat most of the common maladies of man: high blood pressure and cholesterol, diabetes, heart disease, cancer, stroke, Acquired Immunodeficiency Syndrome (AIDS), and more. Taken correctly, the benefits of these medications far outweigh their side effects, though the latter remains a concern even in medications prescribed and taken correctly.

But the growth in medications (there are now more than 10,000 prescription drugs and biologicals—and 300,000 over-the-counter products—available in the United States[1]) has led to a huge increase in the complexity of the medication prescribing and administration process. It has been estimated that at least 5% of hospital patients experience an *adverse drug event* (ADE; harm experienced by a patient as a result of a medication; it can be from a side effect or the consequence of an error) at some point during their hospitalization. Another 5–10% experience a potential ADE, meaning that they almost take the wrong medicine or the wrong dose but don't, often because of a last minute catch or dumb luck.[2] And nearly 1 in 20 hospital admissions can be traced to problems with medications, many of them preventable.[3] Things aren't much safer outside the hospital: when a large group of outpatients on a variety of medications were followed for 3 months, about one in four suffered an ADE, many of them serious.[4]

Although many discussions about medication errors focus on the near-iconic illegibility of physicians' handwriting, two studies have shown that doctors' handwriting is no worse than that of many other professionals,[5, 6] and bad handwriting is an unusual cause of medication errors.

In fact, many steps along the way are vulnerable to mistakes. To illustrate these steps, let's dissect the anatomy of an inpatient prescription (in a hospital without computerized order entry or bar code medication administration):

- A physician handwrites a prescription in the "Doctors' Orders" section of the chart.
- The clerk removes a carbon copy of the order and faxes it to the pharmacy, while a nurse transcribes another copy into the Medication Administration Record (MAR).
- A pharmacist receives the faxed copy, reads it, and retypes the medication, dose, and frequency into the pharmacy's computer system, which generates labels and a bill and helps track inventory.
- The pharmacist manually transfers the medication (if a pill) from a large bottle into "unit-doses"—either cups or a shrink-wrapped container. Intravenous medication may require specialized mixing.
- The medication is delivered to patient's floor; the label includes the name of the medication and the patient's name. The medicine may be delivered on a cart wheeled to the floor, or through a manual transport or pneumatic tube system.
- The nurse goes to the MAR, sees that her patient is due for a medication, searches the medication cart for it, and walks to the patient's room with the medication (along with different medications for her other patients).
- The nurse enters the patient's room, confirms the patient's identity, checks the medication, and administers it.

Believe it or not, I have simplified this process so that it does not take up too much space. Several hospitals have found an average of about *50–100 steps* between a doctor's decision to order a medicine and the delivery of the medicine to the patient. The outpatient process is simpler, but only by a bit. There, the doctor usually gives the patient a paper prescription to carry to a pharmacy. Not only can there be errors in the prescription itself (wrong medicine, wrong dose, illegible prescription, failure to consider allergies or drug-drug, drug-disease, or drug-diet interactions), the administration of the medication (generally a mistake in the pharmacy), or a failure to monitor properly (forgetting to check electrolytes and creatinine in a patient started on a diuretic and angiotensin-converting-enzyme inhibitor), but a new source of errors is added: patients themselves (e.g., failure to follow instructions properly or storing the medications in incorrect bottles).[7] With all these steps, a statistical problem takes its toll: in a 50-step process in which each step is done correctly 99% of the time, the chance that at least one error will occur is a staggering 39%!

Sarah Geller (a pseudonym) was a 68-year-old woman who had undergone a cardiac bypass operation. After a stormy postoperative course she seemed to be on the road to recovery. However, on the morning of her planned transfer out of the intensive care unit (ICU), she suffered a grand mal seizure. This shocked her caregivers: she had no seizure history and was not on any epileptogenic medications. They drew some blood tests, and emergently wheeled her to the computed tomography (CT) scanner to rule out the possibility of a stroke or intracerebral hemorrhage. While she was in transit, the lab paged the doctors to report that Geller's serum glucose was undetectable. Despite multiple infusions of glucose, she never recovered from her coma. In the subsequent investigation, it was determined that her bedside tray in the ICU contained vials of both heparin (used to "flush" her intravenous lines to keep them open) and insulin. The vials were of similar size and shape (Figure 4–2). The nurse, intending to flush Ms. Geller's line with heparin, had inadvertently administered a fatal dose of insulin.[8]

As this case demonstrates, solutions to the problem of medication errors will need to tackle both the prescribing and the administration

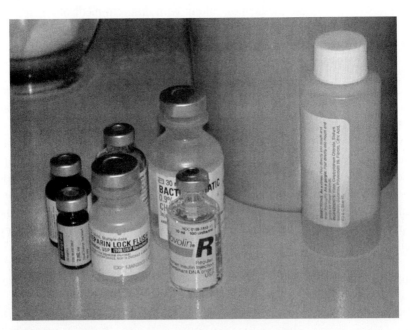

FIGURE 4–2. Heparin and insulin vials on a bedside tray.

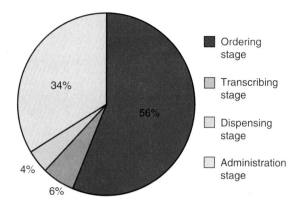

FIGURE 4–3. Medication errors, by stage of the medication process. (Reproduced with permission from Bates DW, Cullen DJ, Laird N, et al. Incidence of adverse drug events and potential adverse drug events. Implications for prevention. ADE Prevention Study Group. *JAMA* 1995;274:29-34.)

phase[1,2] (Figure 4–3). Many of the solutions will be technological: the role of computerized provider order entry (CPOE), computerized decision support, and bar coding and/or radiofrequency identification (RFID) systems will be discussed in Chapter 13. The remainder of this chapter will focus on solutions more specific to the medication prescribing and administration process: standardization, double checks, unit-dosing, removal of medications from certain settings, the role of clinical pharmacists, and meeting the challenges of look-alike, sound-alike medications.

STRATEGIES TO DECREASE MEDICATION ERRORS

Standardization and Decreasing Ambiguity

Betsy Lehman, a popular Boston Globe health columnist, was hospitalized for recurrent breast cancer at Dana-Farber Cancer Institute in 1994. Her experimental protocol called for her to receive an unusually high dose of cyclophosphamide (a chemotherapy agent), followed by a bone marrow transplant. The ordering physicians wrote a prescription: "cyclophosphamide 4 g/sq m over four days," intending that she receive a total of four grams per square meter of body surface area spread out over four days. Instead, the nurses administered the total dose

(4 grams per square meter) on each *of the four days, a fourfold overdose. She died within a month.*

The Lehman case, one of the catalysts for the modern patient safety movement (Table 1–1), can be seen as an argument for computerization and decision support. It would be easy to envision a computer system pre-programmed with the correct dose of chemotherapy that either presented that dose as a default option to the physicians, or automatically alarmed when someone prescribed an out-of-range dose. But the case also screams out for standardization: general agreements on inviolable ways of communicating certain orders that would be understandable to everyone. For example, a hospital could mandate that all medications given over multiple days *must* have the daily dose written each day. Or that high-risk medications could only be ordered one day at a time.

One source of ambiguity has been the long-standing use of abbreviations for certain medications. In 2003, the Joint Commission prohibited hospitals from using a group of "high-risk abbreviations" (Table 4–1),

TABLE 4–1		
The Joint Commission's "Do Not Use" list		
Do not use	**Potential problem**	**Use instead**
U (unit)	Mistaken for "0" (zero), the number "4" (four) or "cc"	Write "unit"
IU (International Unit)	Mistaken for IV (intravenous) or the number 10 (ten)	Write "International Unit"
Q.D., QD, q.d., qd (daily)	Mistaken for each other	Write "daily"
Q.O.D., QOD, q.o.d, qod (every other day)	Period after the Q mistaken for "I" and the "O" mistaken for "I"	Write "every other day"
Trailing zero (X.0 mg) Lack of leading zero (.X mg)	Decimal point is missed	Write X mg Write 0.X mg
MS	Can mean morphine sulfate or magnesium sulfate	Write "morphine sulfate"
MSO_4 and $MgSO_4$	Confused for one another	Write "magnesium sulfate"

Reproduced with permission from http://www.jointcommission.org/PatientSafety/DoNot UseList/

instead insisting that the full name of these medications and instructions ("morphine sulfate," not "MS04", "Insulin 10 Units," not "Insulin 10 U") be spelled out. One of the advantages of CPOE will be to further standardize nomenclature and markedly limit the use of abbreviations. However, as will be further discussed in Chapter 13, CPOE has the capacity to create new classes of medication errors if it is not well designed and implemented.[9,10] For example, unless sophisticated decision support is built into the system, a provider intending to prescribe "penicillin" can easily select the anti-inflammatory agent "penicillamine" from an alphabetical computerized pick list.[11]

Double Checks

Other high-risk industries (nuclear power, aviation, the armed services) have long used double, and even triple checks, to ensure that critical processes are executed correctly. One measure of the relatively low priority healthcare historically gave to patient safety is that until recently the only process in most institutions characterized by standardized and inviolable independent double checks was the blood administration process (in which two nurses checked ABO blood types prior to a transfusion). Thankfully, most hospitals have now built in double checks for chemotherapy and other high-risk medications. However, even when double checks are required by policy, it is critical to ensure that they are truly independent. It is very easy (natural, in fact) for the second check to become lackadaisical, in essence a rubber stamp, thereby providing false reassurance rather than truly increased safety.

Unit-Dosing

This refers to the packaging of medications in ready-to-use units that are prepared in the pharmacy and then delivered to the clinical floor. It was developed in the 1960s, replacing the old method in which the pharmacy sent large bottles of pills or intravenous medications to a floor, expecting that the nurses would perform the mixing or dispensing. Studies have generally found that unit-dose administration is associated with fewer medication errors, and the practice has now become nearly ubiquitous in American hospitals.[12] Many pharmacy systems now include automatic dispensing machines, which are increasingly computerized and linked to centralized inventory control systems.[13]

Removal of Medications from Certain Settings

The most widely cited example of this strategy is the removal of concentrated intravenous potassium from patient care areas. Because of the dangers of potassium overdoses (such as stopping the heart, as when potassium is used as the agent of choice in capital punishment), such removal seems like a good idea. Rather than having the nurses add potassium to their intravenous solutions on the floor, the new system depends on potassium being added to intravenous bags by pharmacists before the premixed bags are sent to the ward.

This approach is an example of a more general strategy called *forcing functions* (Chapters 2 and 7): technical or physical obstacles designed to markedly decrease the probability of error in error-prone circumstances or environments. Forcing functions are designed to anticipate common human errors and try to make harm from them impossible by blocking either the error or its consequences. As mentioned in Chapter 2, the most widely cited example of a forcing function was the reengineering of automobile braking systems in the 1970s to make it impossible to shift a car into reverse when the driver's foot was off the brake.

The removal of concentrated potassium from the medical ward would seem to be such a forcing function, and thus a logical safety solution. The problem is that many nurses found that it took too long for their intravenous drips to arrive from the pharmacy.[14] Because potassium was still allowed in the ICUs (there it often needs to be given emergently), floor nurses began pilfering potassium from ICU stashes and hoarding it, creating an even more chaotic and potentially unsafe situation. The message behind this experience is not that keeping dangerous medications like potassium on the floor is a good idea (it probably isn't), but rather that frontline workers will often thwart apparently "commonsensical safety fixes" when the fixes get in the way of their perceived ability to get their jobs done, a process known as a "workaround."[15] Safety planners need to seek out such actual or potential workarounds through focus groups and observations of providers doing their daily work, lest they create an "underground economy" in unsafe practices (Chapter 7).

The Use of Clinical Pharmacists

Of all the strategies employed to try to decrease medication errors, the insertion of clinical pharmacists into the medication prescribing and administration processes is one of the most powerful (of course, this is in addition to having pharmacists read prescriptions and dispense medications, both core functions). For example, in one study, clinical pharmacists became part of an ICU team in an academic medical center. They educated the physicians and trainees, rounded with the teams, and intervened when they saw a medication error in the making. The intervention resulted in a nearly threefold decrease in the frequency of ADEs, which led to less patient harm and significant cost savings.[16] A more recent study found an even greater reduction (78%) in preventable ADEs when pharmacists rounded with teams on the general medical wards.[17] Unfortunately, in the United States, the high cost and a national shortage of pharmacists has led this strategy to be relatively underemployed.

Meeting the Challenge of Look-Alike, Sound-Alike Medications

Table 4–2 is a list of common medications that have been the subject of sound-alike, look-alike errors. Although the U.S. Food and Drug Administration (FDA) now tries to minimize the possibility that a new medication name will be confused with an old one during its approval process, with 10,000 agents in the pharmacopoeia some problems are inevitable. Among the most confusing examples: the anticonvulsant Cerebyx and the anti-inflammatory Celebrex, the antidepressant Zyprexa and the antihistamine Zyrtec, and the mood stabilizer Lamictal and the antifungal Lamisil. There are a number of strategies to help minimize the risk of confusion, including the user of "tall man" lettering for the suffixes of drugs that begin with the same prefix, like "ClomiPHENE" and "ClomiPRAMINE." But eradicating this problem will require technological help, including bar coding administration systems[18] and computerized order entry with decision support.[19] For example, one can imagine a system that would ask for each medication's indication, and balk if the indication was "seizures" and the chosen medication was Celebrex (instead of Cerebyx) (see Chapter 13).

KEY POINTS

- With the explosive growth in available medications, ADEs (both side effects and medication errors) are one of the most common threats to patient safety.

TABLE 4-2

Medications that have been the subject of sound-alike, look-alike errors

Generic drug names*	Brand names
Acetohexamide/acetazolamide	Adderall/Inderal
Amiodarone/amrinone[†]	Alupent/Atrovent[†]
Bupropion/buspirone	Ambien/Amen
Chlorpromazine/chlorpropamide	Asacol/Os-Cal
Clomiphene/clomipramine	Cardizem/Cardiem
Cyclosporine/cycloserine	Celebrex/Celexa/Cerebyx
Daunorubicin/doxorubicin	Dynacin/DynaCirc
Dimenhydrinate/diphenhydramine	Flomax/Fosamax; Flomax/Volmax
Dobutamine/dopamine[†]	Indinavir/Denavir
Glipizide/glyburide[†]	Lamictal/Lomotil/Lamisil
Hydralazine/hydroxyzine	Lanoxin/Lonox
Methylprednisolone/methyltestosterone	Levbid/Lopid/Lithobid
Nicardipine/nifedipine[†]	Levoxyl/Luvox
Prednisone/prednisolone	Lovenox/Lotronex
Sulfadiazine/sulfisoxazole	Nizoral/Nasarel/Neoral
Tolazamide/tolbutamide	Remeron/Zemuron
Vinblastine/vincristine[†]	Vioxx/Zyvox
	Zyrtec/Zyprexa

[*]In 2001, the U.S. FDA began requiring the manufacturers of many of these products to use "tall man" lettering (e.g., clomiPHENE and clopmiPRAMINE) on their labels. A table that shows these changes appears on the FDA's web site (www.fda.gov).
[†]Drugs have similar action or indication (e.g., glipizide and glyburide are both oral hypoglycemics prescribed to type 2 diabetics).
Reproduced with permission from Cohen MR. The 2-week itch. AHRQ WebM&M (serial online), 2003. Available at: http://webmm. ahrq.gov/case.aspx?caseID=10.

- Errors can occur at any point in the medication use chain, particularly in the prescribing and administration stages. For medications taken in the ambulatory environment, patient-related errors and inadequate monitoring are also common.

- Information technology is likely to decrease medication errors, including prescribing errors (through CPOE and computerized decision support) and administration errors (through bar coding and other identification techniques).

- In addition to these information technology-related solutions, other important safety strategies include: standardization, double checks, unit-dosing, removal of high-risk medications from

certain settings, engaging clinical pharmacists, and specific strategies to mitigate the risks of look-alike, sound-alike medications.

REFERENCES

1. Aspden P, Wolcott J, Bootman JL, et al., eds. Committee on Identifying and
   Preventing Medication Errors. *Preventing Medication Errors: Quality
   Chasm Series*. Institute of Medicine. Washington, DC: The National
   Academy Press, 2007.
2. Bates DW, Cullen DJ, Laird N, et al. Incidence of adverse drug events and
   potential adverse drug events. Implications for prevention. ADE Prevention
   Study Group. *JAMA* 1995;274:29–34.
3. Winterstein AG, Sauer BC, Hepler CD, et al. Preventable drug-related hospital admissions. *Ann Pharmacother* 2002;36:1238–1248.
4. Gandhi TK, Weingart SN, Borus J, et al. Adverse drug events in ambulatory
   care. *N Engl J Med* 2003;348:1556–1564.
5. Berwick DM, Winickoff DE. The truth about doctors' handwriting: a
   prospective study. *BMJ* 1996;313:1657–1658.
6. Schneider KA, Murray CW, Shadduck RD, et al. Legibility of doctors'
   handwriting is as good (or bad) as everyone else's. *Qual Saf Health Care*
   2006;15:445.
7. Shojania KG. Safe medication prescribing and monitoring in the outpatient
   setting. *CMAJ* 2006;174:1257–1258.
8. Bates DW. Unexpected hypoglycemia in a critically ill patient. *Ann Intern
   Med* 2002;137:110–116.
9. Koppel R. What do we know about medication errors made via a CPOE
   system versus those made via handwritten orders? *Crit Care* 2005;
   9:427–428.
10. Han YY, Carcillo JA, Venkataraman ST, et al. Unexpected increased mortal-
    ity after implementation of a commercially sold computerized physician
    order entry system. *Pediatrics* 2005;116:1506–1512. [Erratum in: *Pediatrics*
    2006;117:594.]
11. Flynn EA. A troubling amine. AHRQ WebM&M (serial online), 2006.
    Available at: http://webmm.ahrq.gov/case.aspx?caseID=136.
12. Murray MD, Shojania KG. Unit-dose drug distribution systems. In: Sho-
    jania KG, Duncan BW, McDonald KM, et al., eds. *Making Health Care
    Safer: A Critical Analysis of Patient Safety Practices*. Evidence Report/
    Technology Assessment No. 43, AHRQ Publication No. 01-E058.
    Rockville, MD: Agency for Healthcare Research and Quality, 2001.
13. Murray MD. Automated medication dispensing devices. In: Shojania KG,
    Duncan BW, McDonald KM, et al., eds. *Making Health Care Safer:
    A Critical Analysis of Patient Safety Practices*. Evidence Report/Technol-

ogy Assessment No. 43, AHRQ Publication No. 01-E058. Rockville, MD: Agency for Healthcare Research and Quality, 2001.

14. Cook R, O'Connor M. Potassium chloride's reappearance on the ward: a signal about coupling and failure. National Patient Safety Foundation Listserve. Message dated February 19, 2002. Available at: http://listserv. npsf.org/SCRIPTS/WA-NPSF.EXE ?A2=ind0202&L=patientsafety-l&F= P&S=&P=8463.

15. Spear SJ, Schmidhofer M. Ambiguity and workarounds as contributors to medical error. *Ann Intern Med* 2005;142:627–630.

16. Leape LL, Cullen DJ, Clapp MD, et al. Pharmacist participation on physician rounds and adverse drug events in the intensive care unit. *JAMA* 1999;282:267–270.

17. Kucukarslan SN, Peters M, Mlynarek M, et al. Pharmacists on rounding teams reduce preventable adverse drug events in hospital general medicine units. *Arch Intern Med* 2003;163:2014– 2018.

18. Poon EG. Universal acceptance of computerized physician order entry: what would it take? *J Hosp Med* 2006;1:209–211.

19. Garg AX, Adhikari NK, McDonald H, et al. Effects of computerized clinical decision support systems on practitioner performance and patient outcomes: a systematic review. *JAMA* 2005;293:1223–1238.

ADDITIONAL READINGS

Bates DW, Spell N, Cullen DJ, et al. The costs of adverse drug events in hospitalized patients. *JAMA* 1997;277:307–311.

Cohen MR, ed. *Medication Errors*, 2nd ed. Washington, DC: American Pharmaceutical Association, 2006.

Coleman EA, Smith JD, Raha D, et al. Posthospital medication discrepancies: prevalence and contributing factors. *Arch Intern Med* 2005;165:1842–1847.

Leape LL, Kabcenell A, Gandhi TK, et al. Reducing adverse drug events: lessons from a breakthrough series collaborative. *Jt Comm J Qual Improv* 2000; 26:321–331.

Weingart SN, Wilson RM, Gibberd RW, et al. Epidemiology of medical error. *BMJ* 2000;320:774–777.

CHAPTER FIVE

Surgical Errors

SOME BASIC CONCEPTS AND TERMS

More than 20 million people undergo surgery every year in the United States alone. In the past, surgery could be extremely dangerous, in part because of the risks of direct complications of the surgery itself (bleeding, infection), and in part because of the high risks of anesthesia. Because of major safety improvements in both these areas, surgeries today are extremely safe, and anesthesia-related deaths are rare.[1] Advances in surgery, anesthesia, and postoperative care have led to major declines in mortality in disorders generally treated by surgery, such as diseases of the gallbladder and appendix.[2]

Nevertheless, a number of troubling surgical safety issues persist. This chapter will deal with some of the more problematic issues directly related to surgery: anesthesia-related safety complications, wrong-site and wrong-patient surgery, and retained foreign bodies. Of course, surgery is not immune to medication errors (Chapter 4), diagnostic errors (Chapter 6), teamwork and communication errors (Chapter 9), and nosocomial infections, including surgical site infections (Chapter 10). These issues will be covered in their respective chapters. At this writing, the use of beta-blockers for surgical patients is controversial, and the appropriate patients for this intervention are still being defined.[3] Rather than a detailed discussion of the literature regarding this issue (which will evolve quickly with the publication of ongoing studies), suffice it to say that the general principles surrounding treating targeted patients with proper medications are likely to comport with similar discussions elsewhere in the book (e.g., venous thromboembolism prophylaxis, Chapter 11).

As with medication errors, in which problems from the intervention are grouped under a broad term ("adverse drug events") that includes both errors and side effects (Chapter 4), some surgical complications occur despite impeccable care, while others are caused by errors. Surgeries account for a relatively high percentage of both adverse events and preventable adverse events. For example, one of the major chart review studies of adverse events (the Utah-Colorado study) found that 45% of all adverse events were in surgical patients; of these, 17% resulted from negligence and 17% led to permanent disability. Looked at another way, 3% of patients who underwent a surgery suffered an adverse event, and half of these were preventable.[4]

The field of surgery has always taken the issue of safety extremely seriously. The first efforts to measure complications of care and approach them scientifically were developed by Boston surgeon Ernest Codman in the early twentieth century. Codman's "End-Result Hospital"—following every patient for evidence of errors in treatment and disseminating the results of this inquiry—was both revolutionary and highly controversial[5-7] (Appendix III). Nevertheless, the American College of Surgeons soon began inspecting hospitals (in 1918), an effort that later served as the nidus for the formation of the Joint Commission (Chapter 20). More recently, the person most responsible for putting safety on the radar screen of modern medicine was another surgeon, Dr. Lucian Leape.[8,9] Despite these remarkable contributions, surgery, like the rest of medicine, has traditionally approached safety as a matter of individual performance: a complication was deemed to represent a failing by the surgeon. Our new focus on systems issues is allowing surgery to make tremendous strides in improving safety.

VOLUME-OUTCOME RELATIONSHIPS

Beginning with a 1979 study by Luft and colleagues that demonstrated a relationship between higher volumes and better outcomes for certain surgeries, a substantial literature has generally supported the commonsensical notion that "practice makes perfect" when it comes to procedures.[10] The precise mechanism for this relationship has not been elucidated, but it seems to hold for both the volume of individual operators (e.g., the surgeon, the interventional cardiologist) as well as the institution (e.g., the hospital or surgicenter).

Although much of the volume-outcome relationship probably owes to the fact that well-functioning teams take time to gel—learning to anticipate each others' reactions and preferences—there also seems to be a learning curve for procedural competence. One of the best-studied examples is that of laparoscopic cholecystectomy, a technique that essentially replaced the more dangerous and costly open cholecystectomy in the early 1990s. As "lap choley" emerged as the preferred procedure for gall-bladder removal, tens of thousands of practicing surgeons needed to learn the procedure well after the completion of their formal training, providing an organic test of the volume-outcome curve.

The findings were sobering. One early study of lap choleys showed that injuries to the common bile duct dropped almost 20-fold once surgeons had at least a dozen cases under their belts.[11] After that, the learning curve flattened, but not by much: the rate of common bile duct injury on the 30th case was still 10 times higher than the rate seen after 50 cases.

One can assume that most graduates of today's surgical residencies are well trained in the techniques of laparoscopic surgery. But in the early days of a new procedure, patients have no such reassurance. A 1991 survey found that only 45% of 165 practicing surgeons who had participated in a 2-day practical course on laparoscopic cholecystectomy felt the workshop had left them adequately prepared to start performing the procedure. Yet three-quarters of these surgeons reported that they implemented the new procedure immediately after returning to their practices.[12]

Obviously, part of the solution to the volume-outcome and the learning curve conundrums will lie in new training models, including the use of realistic simulation (Chapter 17). Some surgical and procedural special-ties are now requiring minimum volumes for privileging and board certifi-cation, and a major coalition of payers (the Leapfrog Group) promotes high volume centers as one of its safety standards under the banner of "evidence-based hospital referral" (Table 5–1). Certain states or insurers are insisting on minimum volumes or channeling patients to higher volume providers (institutions that achieve good outcomes and have high volumes are sometimes dubbed "Centers of Excellence").

Although such policies appear attractive at first, they carry several risks. First, patients may not be anxious to travel long distances to receive care from high volume providers or institutions. Second, at some point high volumes may actually compromise quality (if they overtax institutions or physicians). Finally, many of the procedures being discussed, such as car-diac or transplant surgery, are relatively lucrative. Their removal could threaten the economic viability of low volume institutions, which often cross-subsidize nonprofitable services (care of the uninsured, trauma care) with profits from the well-reimbursed surgeries.

All of this is not to say that channeling patients to high volume (or better yet, demonstrably safer or higher quality[13]) doctors and practices is a mis-take, but rather that it is a complex maneuver that requires thoughtful con-sideration of both expected and unforeseen consequences.

TABLE 5–1

The Leapfrog Group's Volume Standards*

Treatment or procedure	Recommended annual volumes: hospitals/surgeons
Coronary artery bypass graft	≥450/100
Percutaneous coronary intervention	≥400/75
Aortic valve replacement	≥120/22
Bariatric surgery	≥100/20
Abdominal aortic aneurysm repair	≥50/22
Esophagectomy	≥13/2
Pancreatic resection	≥11/2
High-risk delivery (expected birth weight <1500 g, gestational age <32 weeks, or prenatal diagnosis of major congenital anomaly)	Neonatal ICU with average daily census ≥15

*Since 2003, The Leapfrog Group added selected process and outcome measures to the minimum volume requirements cited above.
Reproduced with permisison from http://www.leapfroggroup.org/media/file/Leapfrog-Evidence-Based_Hospital_Referral_Fact_Sheet.pdf.

PATIENT SAFETY IN ANESTHESIA

Although it is often stated that the modern patient safety movement began in late 1999 with the publication of *To Err is Human*,[14] the field of anesthesia is a noteworthy exception. Anesthesia began focusing on safety a generation earlier, and its success story holds lessons for the rest of the patient safety field.

In 1972, a young engineer named Jeff Cooper began work at the Anesthesia Bioengineering Unit at Massachusetts General Hospital (MGH), unsure of his future. Like Codman 60 years earlier, what he saw at MGH bothered him—mistakes were common, cover-ups were the norm, and systems to prevent errors were glaringly absent. Even worse, many procedures and environments appeared to be all-but-designed to promote errors. For example, he noticed that turning the dial clockwise increased the dose of anesthetic in some anesthesia machines, and decreased it in others. Soon thereafter, Cooper delivered a lecture entitled "The Anesthesia Machine: An Accident Waiting to Happen." He and colleagues soon began looking at procedures and equipment through a human factors lens (Chapter 7), using the technique of "critical incident analysis" to explore all causative factors for mistakes.[15–17]

At the same time, anesthesiology was in the midst of a malpractice crisis characterized by terrific acrimony and skyrocketing premiums. Several other researchers, recognizing the possibility that there might be error patterns, began carefully reviewing settled malpractice cases for themes and lessons ("closed-case analysis").[18] And they found them, in the form of poor machine design, lack of standardization, lax policies and procedures, poor education, and more.

The research and insights from Cooper's work and the closed-case analyses were important, but they needed to be brought into the mainstream, particularly among physicians. Luckily, as so often happens, the right person emerged at the right time. Ellison Pierce, known to all as "Jeep," assumed the presidency of the American Society of Anesthesiologists in 1983. Pierce, energized in part by the experience of a friend's daughter, who died under anesthesia during a routine dental procedure, conceived of a foundation to help support work to make care safer—in fact, he probably coined the term "patient safety" in founding the Anesthesia Patient Safety Foundation (APSF). APSF, working closely with other professional groups, healthcare organizations, and industry, helped push the field to new heights, beginning by convincing caregivers that there was a real problem and that it was soluble with the right approach.[19]

What lessons from anesthesia are relevant to the rest of our efforts to improve patient safety?[1,20,21] First, patient safety requires strong leadership, with a commitment to openness and a willingness to embrace change. Second, learning from past mistakes is a vital part of patient safety efforts. In the case of anesthesia, the closed-case reviews led to key insights. Third, although technology is not the complete answer to safety, it must be a part of the answer. In anesthesia, the thoughtful application of oximetry, capnography, and automated blood pressure monitoring have been vital. Fourth, where applicable, the use of human factors engineering and forcing functions can be key adjuncts to safety (Chapter 7). For example, the often-cited example of changing the anesthesia tubing so that the incorrect gasses could not be hooked up was crucial; this was a far more effective maneuver than trying to educate or remind anesthesiologists about the possibility of mix-ups. Finally, anesthesia was in the throes of both a malpractice crisis and a number of highly visible errors in the media. Sparks like these are often necessary to disrupt the inertia and denial that sabotage so many safety efforts. The fact that malpractice rates for anesthesiologists, which had been among the highest among medical specialties in the mid-1980s, are now in the midrange of all specialties (in large part because errors that cause patient harm have become so unusual) raises hope that there may truly be a "business case for safety."

WRONG-SITE/WRONG-PATIENT SURGERY

In 1995, Willie King, a 51-year-old diabetic man with severe peripheral vascular disease, checked into a hospital in Tampa, Florida for amputation of a gangrenous right leg. The admitting clerk mistakenly entered into the computer system that Mr. King was there for a left below-the-knee amputation. An alert floor nurse caught the error after seeing a printout of the day's operating room (OR) schedule; she called the OR to correct the mistake. A scrub nurse made a handwritten correction to the printed schedule, but the computer's schedule was not changed. Since this computer schedule was the source of subsequent printed copies, copies of the incorrect schedule were distributed around the OR and hospital. King's surgeon entered the OR, read the wrong procedure off one of the printed schedules, prepped the wrong leg, and then began to amputate it. The error was discovered partway through the surgery, too late to save the left leg. Of course, the gangrenous right leg still needed to be removed. A few weeks later it was, leaving King a double amputee.

Events like these are so egregious that they have been dubbed "Never Events"—meaning that they should never occur under any circumstances (Appendix VI). And who could possibly disagree. When one hears of cases like this, it is also difficult to resist the instinct to assign blame, usually to the surgeon who operated on the wrong body part. Yet we know that such events are sufficiently common—in one survey of approximately 1000 hand surgeons, 20% admitted to having operated on the wrong site at least once in their career, and an additional 16% had prepared to operate on the wrong site but caught themselves before the moment of truth—that there must be something more than simply a careless surgeon or nurse at play.[22] And the answer, as usual, is Swiss cheese (Chapter 2) and bad systems. Appreciating this makes clear the need for multidimensional solutions that aim to decrease the holes in each layer of Swiss cheese and create multiple overlapping layers to block inevitable human slips from causing terrible harm.

The Joint Commission has promoted the use of the *Universal Protocol* to prevent wrong-site and wrong-patient surgery and procedures (Table 5–2). In essence, the Protocol acknowledges that single solutions to this problem are destined to fail, and that robust fixes depend on multiple overlapping layers of protection. A couple of the elements of the Universal Protocol merit further comment. At first glance, *sign-your-site*—the surgeon marks the surgical site in indelible ink after verifying the correct site—would appear to be a particularly strong solution. But the early history of sign-your-site demonstrates that even reasonable safety solutions are destined to fail without strong standard policies and enforcement protocols. In the mid-1990s, before the Joint Commission or surgical professional societies entered the fray, a number of well-meaning orthopedic surgeons began to use markings to help ensure that they operated on the correct surgical site. Unfortunately, without a standardized approach, the result was inevitable: some surgeons placed an "X" on the surgical site (as in, "X marks the spot"), while others placed an "X" on the *opposite* limb (as in "don't cut here"). Although there were no documented cases of wrong-site surgery resulting from this anarchy, the implementation of standard rules was crucial (under the Universal Protocol, the surgical site is the only one to be marked).

TABLE 5–2

The Joint Commission's "Universal Protocol for preventing wrong-site, wrong-procedure, and wrong-person surgery"

Preoperative verification process

Process: An ongoing process of information gathering and verification, beginning with the determination to do the procedure, continuing through all settings and interventions involved in the preoperative preparation of the patient, up to and including the "time out" just before the start of the procedure.

Marking the operative site

Process: For procedures involving right/left distinction, multiple structures (such as fingers and toes), or multiple levels (as in spinal procedures), the intended site must be marked such that the mark will be visible after the patient has been prepped and draped.

"Time out" immediately before starting the procedure

Process: Active communication among all members of the surgical/procedure team, consistently initiated by a designated member of the team, conducted in a "fail-safe" mode, i.e., the procedure is not started until any questions or concerns are resolved.

Reproduced with permission from The Joint Commission. Available at: http://www.jointcommission.org/NR/rdonlyres/E3C600EB-043B-4E86-B04E-CA4A89AD5433/0/ universal_protocol.pdf.

Another key element in the Universal Protocol is the *time out*, during which the entire surgical team is supposed to huddle and then briefly discuss and agree upon the patient's name and intended procedure. This too seems like a robust safety solution, a fail-safe step that is sure to catch any errors that eluded prior protections. Yet we have come to recognize how dependent this step is on having a culture of safety (Chapters 9 and 15), one in which people low in the hierarchy are comfortable raising their concerns "up the authority gradient." Without a safety culture and good communication, interventions such as time outs can be robotic and perfunctory, providing the illusion, rather than the reality, of safety.[23]

RETAINED SPONGES AND INSTRUMENTS

In October 2002, a Canadian woman repeatedly tripped the alarm on a metal detector as she attempted to board a flight in Regina, Saskatchewan. On a closer search, the detector wand continued to bleep as it was passed over her abdomen. Since security personnel were unable to identify anything metallic on her person, they let her board her flight to Calgary. The woman wondered whether the episode was related to the recurrent stomach pain she'd been experiencing ever since her abdominal surgery four months earlier. After her trip, she saw her doctor, who ordered an abdominal x-ray. Shockingly, it showed the outline of metal retractor, a tool used by the surgical team months earlier. The surgeons had inadvertently left the object behind when they closed up, which was no small feat—the retractor was a foot long and two inches wide, practically the size of a crowbar.

The term "retained sponge" is often used as a catchall phrase for all manner of surgical paraphernalia left behind after surgery. A review by Gawande of 54 patients with retained foreign bodies over a 16-year period found that roughly two-thirds were actual sponges—square or rectangular bits of absorbent gauze designed to soak up blood in the operative field—while the remaining third were surgical instruments.[24] This frequency corresponds to an overall "retained sponge" rate of about 1 per 10,000 surgeries, which works out to at least one case each year for a typical large hospital in the United States. Because the study drew its sample from malpractice cases, the problem is undoubtedly more common than this published estimate.

Unlike many other safety problems, the retained sponge/instrument problem would seem to be preventable by the thoughtful implementation of systematic, mechanical solutions. In the 1940s, manufacturers produced sponges with loops that were attached to a 2-in. metal ring. The ring then hung outside the operative field while the sponges were placed inside the field. When the operation was over, the nurse simply harvested the sponges by gathering the rings—the way a trail of fishing hooks is pulled out of the water by reeling in the line. Clever as this sounds, surgeons found the ring system unwieldy, and many simply cut the rings off: a classic example of a *routine rule violation*. By the 1960s, manufacturers tried another approach, producing surgical sponges with an embedded radiopaque thread (Figure 5–1a) meant to show up on x-rays (Figure 5–1b). But obtaining a postoperative x-ray on every patient is impractical, so the x-ray solution usually comes into play months later, when a patient has persistent postoperative pain and the doctors are trying to figure out why.

To laypeople, leaving a sponge or tool behind may seem like a particularly boneheaded error–until you remember that complex or emergency surgeries often require dozens, even hundreds, of sponges (along with scores of other instruments and needles), often placed under considerable time pressure. This is one reason surgical teams have long used "sponge, sharp, and instrument counts." The standard protocol requires four separate counts: when the instruments are set up and the sponges are unpacked, when the surgery begins and the items are called for and used, at the time of closure, and finally during external suturing. Unfortunately, the chaotic and pressured circumstances in most busy operating rooms (ORs), coupled with the reluctance of the nurses to admit (consciously or not) to the fallacy of an earlier count, creates situations in which the counts fail. In Gawande's most startling finding, while one-third of the retained sponge cases had not been subject to a documented count, two-thirds of the cases were.[24] And in about half the cases, there were actually *multiple counts documented to be in agreement*. This means that every sponge and instrument was accounted for, despite the fact that one would turn up later— rather inconveniently—in a patient's abdomen.

The real lesson from all of this is that what appears to be a perfectly logical safety practice often turns out to be highly imperfect. Because sponge counts of any kind are inherently unreliable, some experts have recommended taking an x-ray of every surgical site before the field is sutured. Even if x-rays were free and patients and staff were willing to put up with the procedure, keeping anesthetized OR patients on the table any longer than strictly necessary creates its own problems. Partly for this

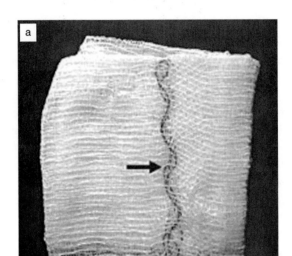

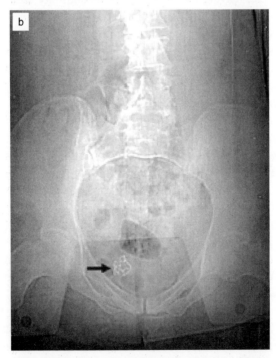

FIGURE 5–1. Surgical sponge (panel a) with an embedded radiopaque thread, shown on x-ray (panel b).

reason, Gawande and his colleagues recommend x-rays only in high-risk cases: those involving emergency surgery, prolonged surgery, surgery involving a real-time change in clinical strategy, and surgery on obese patients. Even this plan is imperfect, because radiopaque markers are subtle and can be easily overlooked on x-rays.

Ultimately, the best solution to the retained sponge problem probably lies in new technology. Some companies are developing sponges embedded with tags that cause a detector-wand to *beep* when the surgeon waves it over the field before closure.[25] Others are working on automatic "sponge counters," like tollbooth coin machines, that can be loaded up and checked after every surgery. It seems likely that one or several of these solutions will be ready for widespread implementation soon, hopefully rendering these errors a historical curiosity.

KEY POINTS

- Patient safety issues in surgery include those common to other fields (e.g., medication errors, nosocomial infections, communication mishaps), but also several specific to surgery (e.g., wrong-site surgery, retained sponges).

- Evidence for a volume-outcome relationship in many surgical areas argues for new types of simulator training.

- Anesthesia embraced the importance of many patient safety principles (systems thinking, human factors engineering, learning from mistakes, standardization) earlier than any other field in medicine, and has amassed the most impressive safety record.

- Systematic application of the "Universal Protocol" (including "sign-your-site" and the preprocedural "time out") is presently the best strategy to prevent wrong-site and wrong-patient errors.

- Retained sponges and other surgical instruments is an uncommon safety hazard. Sponge counts and x-rays are presently the main preventative strategies, but prevention will ultimately depend on more robust detection technologies.

REFERENCES

1. Gaba DM. Anaesthesiology as a model for patient safety in health care. *BMJ* 2000;320:785–788.
2. Milamed DR, Hedley-Whyte J. Contributions of the surgical sciences to a reduction of the mortality rate in the United States for the period 1968 to 1988. *Ann Surg* 1994;219:94–102.
3. Lindenauer PK, Pekow P, Wang K, et al. Perioperative beta-blocker therapy and mortality after major noncardiac surgery. *N Engl J Med* 2005; 353:349–361.
4. Thomas EJ, Studdert DM, Burstin HR, et al. Incidence and types of adverse events and negligent care in Utah and Colorado. *Med Care* 2000;38:261–271.
5. Sharpe VA, Faden AI. *Medical Harm: Historical, Conceptual and Ethical Dimensions of Iatrogenic Illness.* Cambridge, England: Cambridge University Press, 1998.
6. Neuhauser D. John Williamson and the terrifying results of the medical practice information demonstration project. *Qual Saf Health Care* 2002;11:387–389.
7. Vincent C. *Patient Safety.* London: Elsevier, 2006.
8. Leape LL. Error in medicine. *JAMA* 1994;272:1851–1857.
9. Leape LL. An interview with Lucian Leape. *Jt Comm J Qual Saf* 2004; 30:653–658.
10. Luft HS, Bunker JP, Enthoven AC. Should operations be regionalized? The empirical relation between surgical volume and mortality. *N Engl J Med* 1979;301:1364–1369.
11. Moore MJ, Bennett CL. The learning curve for laparoscopic cholecystectomy. The Southern Surgeons Club. *Am J Surg* 1995;170:55–59.
12. Morino M, Festa V, Garrone C. Survey on Torino courses. The impact of a two-day practical course on apprenticeship and diffusion of laparoscopic cholecystectomy in Italy. *Surg Endosc* 1995;9:46–48.
13. Shahian DM. Improving cardiac surgery quality—volume, outcome, process? *JAMA* 2004;291:246–248.
14. Kohn L, Corrigan J, Donaldson M, eds. *To Err is Human: Building a Safer Health System.* Washington, DC: Committee on Quality of Health Care in America, Institute of Medicine: National Academy Press, 2000.
15. Cooper JB, Newbower RS, Long CD, et al. Preventable anesthesia mishaps: a study of human factors. *Anesthesiology* 1978;49:399–406.
16. Cooper JB, Long CD, Newbower RS, et al. Critical incidents associated with intraoperative exchanges of anesthesia personnel. *Anesthesiology* 1982;56:456–461.
17. Cooper JB, Newbower RS, Kitz RJ. An analysis of major errors and equipment failures in anesthesia management: considerations for prevention and detection. *Anesthesiology* 1984;60:34–42.

18. Caplan RA, Posner KL, Ward RJ, et al. Adverse respiratory events in anesthesia: a closed claims analysis. *Anesthesiology* 1990;72:828–833.
19. Gawande A. *Complications: A Surgeon's Notes on an Imperfect Science.* New York, NY: Metropolitan Books, 2002.
20. Lagasse RS. Anesthesia safety: model or myth? A review of the published literature and analysis of current original data. *Anesthesiology* 2002; 97:1609–1617.
21. Cooper JB. Getting into patient safety: a personal story. AHRQ WebM&M (serial online), August 2006. Available at: http://webmm. ahrq.gov/perspective.aspx?perspectiveID=29
22. Meinberg EG, Stern PJ. Incidence of wrong-site surgery among hand surgeons. *J Bone Joint Surg Am* 2003;85-A(2):193–197.
23. Seiden SC, Barach P. Wrong-side/wrong-site, wrong-procedure, and wrong-patient adverse events: are they preventable? *Arch Surg* 2006; 141:931–939.
24. Gawande AA, Studdert DM, Oray EJ, et al. Risk factors for retained instruments and sponges after surgery. *N Engl J Med* 2003;348:229–235.
25. Macario A, Morris D, Morris S. Initial evaluation of a handheld device for detecting retained surgical gauze sponges using radiofrequency identification technology. *Arch Surg* 2006;141:659–662.

ADDITIONAL READINGS

Bosk CL. *Forgive and Remember: Managing Medical Failure,* 2nd ed. Chicago, IL: University of Chicago Press, 2003.

Carthey J, de Leval MR, Reason JT. The human factor in cardiac surgery: errors and near misses in a high technology medical domain. *Ann Thorac Surg* 2001;72:300–305.

Gawande A. *Better: A Surgeon's Notes on Performance.* New York, NY: Metropolitan Books, 2007.

Makary MA, Sexton JB, Freischlag JA, et al. Patient safety in surgery. *Ann Surg* 2006;243:628–635.

Michaels RK, Makary MA, Dehab Y, et al. Achieving the National Quality Forum's "Never Events": prevention of wrong site, wrong procedure, and wrong patient operations. *Ann Surg* 2007;245:526–532.

Pierce EC. 40 years behind the mask: safety revisited. *Anesthesiology* 1996;29:965–975.

Sexton JB, Makary MA, Tersigni AR, et al. Teamwork in the operating room; frontline perspectives among hospitals and operating room personnel. *Anesthesiology* 2006;105:877–884.

CHAPTER SIX

Diagnostic Errors

SOME BASIC CONCEPTS AND TERMS

The modern patient safety movement has emphasized medication errors, handoff errors, infections, and surgical errors; all areas amenable to technological (e.g., computerized order entry), procedural (e.g., double checks), and policy (e.g., "sign-your-site") solutions. Diagnostic errors have been less well emphasized, in part because they are more difficult to measure and to fix.

Yet a number of studies have demonstrated that diagnostic errors are common, and that they can be deadly.[1,2] At first glance, diagnostic errors would seem to represent human failings—pure failures of cognition. And it is true that, perhaps more than any other area in the field of patient safety, the training and skills of the diagnostician remains of paramount importance. However, in keeping with our modern understanding of patient safety, there are systems fixes that can decrease their frequency and consequences.

MISSED MYOCARDIAL INFARCTION: A CLASSIC DIAGNOSTIC ERROR

Annie Jackson (names are pseudonyms), a 68-year-old African-American woman with mild diabetes, high blood pressure, and elevated cholesterol presented to the emergency department after 30 minutes of squeezing chest discomfort. An ECG was quickly obtained. The ER physician, Dr. Bennett, studied the tracing and saw some nonspecific changes in the ST and T segments—not entirely normal but not the ST-segment elevations that are classic for acute myocardial infarction (MI). On exam, he found mild tachycardia, clear lungs, and mild tenderness over the lower part of the patient's sternum. He considered the latter discovery quite reassuring (after all, such tenderness would be more characteristic of a musculoskeletal process than a heart attack), but also ordered a troponin (a biomarker released by damaged heart cells). It came back mildly elevated, again not in the range specific for MI but not normal either. Nevertheless, he made a diagnosis of costochondritis (inflammation of the sternum-rib joint), prescribed an anti-inflammatory agent and bed rest, and released Ms. Jackson from the emergency department. She died later that night, a victim of an untreated MI.

We can only guess which cognitive error caused Dr. Bennett to release Annie Jackson from the ER. Perhaps because she was a woman, he underestimated her chance of having a heart attack. He almost certainly relied too heavily on chest wall tenderness for his diagnosis—it is unusual, but not unheard of, in MI patients. He also overemphasized the lack of clear evidence on the ECG and troponin tests. Although they were "nonspecific," both were clearly abnormal and thus justified admission. Maybe he was just exhausted after a long day at work.

We do know, however, that this particular error—sending patients home with heart attacks—is distressingly common and frequently lethal. Nearly 1 in 25 patients with MIs are mistakenly sent home, and these patients have a much higher death rate than MI victims who are correctly diagnosed and hospitalized. Because the diagnosis of missed MI is the best-studied diagnostic error, I will use it to make several broader points about these errors.

Researchers studying the problem of missed MIs quickly concluded that many errors were related to patient demographics. Physicians were more likely to send patients home despite worrisome histories or abnormal data when the patients were in groups traditionally believed to be at lower risk for MI, such as women and those under age 55. Nonwhites were also mistakenly sent home more often, raising the question of racial bias, conscious or unconscious, among caregivers.[3] In one particularly sobering study, 720 physicians were shown videotapes of actors playing patients with chest pain that could have been heart related.[4] Four actors, each speaking precisely the same script, appeared on the videos: a white man, a white woman, a black man, and a black woman. Regardless of their own race and ethnicity, the physicians were far more likely to recommend cardiac catheterization for the white male than for the black female. Similar variations in diagnostic and therapeutic practices have been seen elsewhere in medicine, catalyzing vigorous efforts to understand and abolish these "healthcare disparities."[5]

Researchers found that physician-specific differences were also at play. For example, one study showed that senior physicians were significantly more likely than their younger colleagues to correctly hospitalize chest pain patients (those with real MIs).[6] Were the older physicians better diagnosticians? Perhaps not—the older physicians were also more likely to hospitalize patients *without* heart attacks. In other words, with experience came risk aversion. Another study showed that risk aversion was not simply a function of age. One-hundred nineteen physicians completed a questionnaire assessing their attitudes toward risk. Doctors who appeared to be risk seekers (e.g., those who like fast cars and sky diving) were four times more likely to send the same chest pain patient home than the risk avoiders.[7]

One could easily look at cases like Annie Jackson's and see careless doctoring, a blown diagnosis, and a fatal mistake. But by now, hopefully, you're approaching this case with a more systems-focused mindset, thinking: How can we improve our ability to diagnose patients who come to the ER with a constellation of symptoms, findings, and risk factors that often yield ambiguous results but can be life-threatening? Too often, without a more systematic approach, the clinical decision—to admit or discharge the patient—is based on the physician's faulty reasoning, which may be traced to poor training, inadequate experience, personal and professional bias, fuzzy thinking brought on by overwork and fatigue, or even the physician's own tolerance for risk.

COGNITIVE ERRORS: ITERATIVE HYPOTHESIS TESTING, BAYESIAN REASONING, AND HEURISTICS

As cognitive psychologists began to study how physicians think, they found that even well-trained doctors can engage in faulty thinking because they take cognitive shortcuts, reinforced by a professional culture that rewards the appearance of certainty over its reality.[8] This means that fixing diagnostic errors is likely to depend on understanding how physicians think about diagnoses, and providing them with tools (either cognitive or adjunctive, such as information technology) to help them make correct decisions more often.

Beginning in the 1970s, several researchers began to try to understand how great diagnosticians think. Led by Dr. Jerome Kassirer (later the editor of the *New England Journal of Medicine*), they observed the diagnostic reasoning of dozens of clinicians, and found that the good ones naturally engaged in a process called *iterative hypothesis testing*. This means that, after hearing the initial portion of a case, they immediately began thinking about possible scenarios to explain the facts, modifying their opinions as more information became available. For example, a skilled physician presented with the case of a 57-year-old man with 3 days of chest pain, shortness of breath, and light-headedness, responds by thinking, "The worst thing this could be is a heart attack or blood clot to the lungs. I need to ask a few more questions to see if the chest pain bores through to the back, which would make me worry about an aortic dissection. I'll also ask about typical cardiac symptoms, such as sweating and nausea, and see if the pain is squeezing or radiates to the left arm or jaw. But even if it doesn't, I'll certainly get an ECG to be sure no cardiac event has occurred. If he also reports a fever or cough, I might begin to suspect pneumonia or pleurisy. The chest x-ray should help sort that out."

Every answer the patient gives and each positive or negative finding on the physical examination (yes, there is a fever; no, the spleen is not enlarged) triggers an automatic, almost intuitive recalibration of the probability of the various alternatives. The skilled diagnostician does this so effortlessly that novices often struggle as they try to understand the science that underlies the expert's decision to embrace certain facts (the clear lung fields in the patient with dyspnea markedly elevates the probability of pulmonary embolism) while discarding others (the absence of an S_3 gallop does little to dissuade the expert from the possibility of heart failure).

We now recognize that much of this art consists of applying an unconscious, intuitive version of *Bayes' theorem*, developed by the eighteenth-century British theologian-turned-mathematician Thomas Bayes. In essence, Bayes' theorem says that any medical test must be interpreted from two perspectives. The first: How accurate is the test?—that is, how often does it give right or wrong answers. The second: How likely is it that this patient has the disease the test is looking for? Bayesian reasoning is why it is foolish to screen apparently healthy 35-year-old executives with a cardiac treadmill test (or, for that matter, a "heart scan"), because positive results will mostly be false positives. Conversely, a 65-year-old smoker with high cholesterol who develops squeezing chest pain when shoveling snow has about a 95% chance of having significant coronary artery disease. In this case, a negative treadmill test only lowers this probability to about 80%, so the clinician who reassures the patient that the normal treadmill means his heart is fine is making a terrible, and potentially fatal, mistake.

In addition to misapplications of iterative hypothesis testing and failure to appreciate the implications of Bayesian reasoning, we now understand that many diagnostic errors are caused by cognitive shortcuts ("heuristics") that clinicians take, often in the name of efficiency. For example, many errors occur when clinicians are too quick to pronounce judgment, and then defend that turf too vigorously when contradictory evidence emerges. This is human nature, of course; we tend to see what we expect to see rather than than what's actually in front of our eyes. By the way, did you notice the word "than" used twice in a row in the previous sentence? Even when we don't intend to do it, our brains can take cognitive shortcuts to get us to our goal—whether it's finishing a sentence or discharging a patient from the ER.

This cognitive bias, known as "anchoring," is only one of the many pitfalls that underlie many diagnostic errors. Others common biases include the availability heuristic, framing effects, blind obedience, and premature closure (Table 6–1).

IMPROVING DIAGNOSTIC REASONING

In Chapter 13, we will explore the role of computerized decision support and more general use of information technology in helping physicians to be better diagnosticians. At this juncture, suffice it to say that such computerized adjuncts are likely to help clinicians make better, more evidence-based decisions, but will not for the foreseeable future replace the clinician's mind as the main diagnostic workhorse.

Can our cognitive biases be overcome? Perhaps more than any area in clinical medicine, when diagnosing patients we need to learn from our mistakes and to deepen our understanding of clinical reasoning. As with most errors, the answer will come through systems thinking, but here this means better systems for training physicians to avoid common diagnostic speed bumps (Table 6–1). As Canadian safety expert and emergency medicine physician Pat Croskerry puts it:

> One uniquely distinguishing characteristic of those who make high-quality decisions is that they can largely free themselves from the common pitfalls to which novices are vulnerable. A rite of passage in all disciplines of medicine is learning about clinical pitfalls that have been identified by the discipline's experts. This [says] in effect, "Here is a typical error that will be made, and here is how to avoid it."[9]

TABLE 6–1

Selected cognitive biases leading to missed diagnoses, and corrective strategies

Circumstance and pitfall	Classic definition	Corrective strategies	Clinical maxims
Availability heuristic	Judging by ease of recalling past cases	Verify with legitimate statistics	Pay attention to base rates: "If you hear hoof beats, think about horses, not zebras."
Anchoring heuristic	Relying on initial impressions	Reconsider in light of new data or second opinion	Think beyond the most favored: "If the patient dies unexpectedly, what would it be from?"
Framing effects	Being swayed by subtle wording	Examine case from alternative perspectives	Deliberately consider from another angle: "Let's play devil's advocate …"
Blind obedience	Showing undue deference to authority or technology	Reconsider when authority is more remote	Tactfully reconfirm human work (in case of human authority); assess test accuracy (in case of technology)
Premature closure	Espousing narrow-minded belief in single idea	Return to case when refreshed (if clinical pace allows)	Give consideration to extremes: "What's the diagnosis that I don't want to miss?"

Reproduced with permission from Redelmeier DA. Improving patient care. The cognitive psychology of missed diagnoses. *Ann Intern Med* 2005;142:115–120.

Interestingly, in the case of the chest pain triage decision (a decision that early researchers hoped to perfect through a combination of electronic decision support and a better appreciation of diagnostic pitfalls), most experts have concluded that the quest for diagnostic certainty is futile. In a number of research studies, even the best algorithms could not reliably identify patients whose actual risk of MI was so low that it was safe to send them home—especially when the penalty for even occasional failure can be a tragic death and a multimillion-dollar lawsuit. So the real progress in chest pain triage has come not from honing our diagnostic abilities, but rather from developing new ways (usually involving repeated cardiac biomarker tests and a predischarge treadmill test) to "rule out MI" inexpensively over a reasonably short (6–12 hours) observational period.[10] In essence, we have abandoned our quest for diagnostic perfection and accepted instead the more mundane task of managing our uncertainty safely by resolving it quickly and inexpensively.

KEY POINTS

- Despite advances in laboratory testing, clinical imaging, and information technology, diagnostic errors remain commonplace.
- Clinicians' diagnostic and therapeutic actions are influenced by both patient-related (e.g., age, gender, race) and clinician-related (e.g., past experience, risk tolerance) factors.
- Good diagnosticians correctly apply iterative hypothesis testing and Bayesian reasoning, and avoid cognitive pitfalls and biases, such as anchoring (getting stuck on initial impressions) and the availability heuristic (being unduly influenced by prior cases).
- Improving diagnostic reasoning will involve both computerized decision support and training clinicians to be more effective and evidence-based diagnostic thinkers.

REFERENCES

1. Shojania KG. Changes in rates of autopsy-detected diagnostic errors over time: a systematic review. *JAMA* 2003;289:2849–2856.
2. Croskerry P. The importance of cognitive errors in diagnosis and strategies to minimize them. *Acad Med* 2003;78:775–780.

3. Lee TH, Rouan GW, Weisberg MC, et al. Clinical characteristics and natural history of patients with acute myocardial infarction sent home from the emergency room. *Am J Cardiol* 1987;60:219–224.

4. Schulman KA, Berlin JA, Harless W, et al. The effect of race and sex on physicians' recommendations for cardiac catheterization. *N Engl J Med* 1999;340:618–626.

5. *National Healthcare Disparities Report: Summary.* Rockville, MD: Agency for Healthcare Research and Quality, February 2004. Available at: http://www.ahrq.gov/qual/nhdr03/nhdrsum03.htm.

6. Ting HH, Lee TH, Soukup JR, et al. Impact of physician experience on triage of emergency room patients with acute chest pain at three teaching hospitals. *Am J Med* 1991;91:401–408.

7. Pearson SD, Goldman L, Orav EJ, et al. Triage decisions for emergency department patients with chest pain: do physicians' risk attitudes make the difference? *J Gen Intern Med* 1995;10:557–564.

8. Friedman CP, Gatti GG, Franz TM, et al. Do physicians know when their diagnoses are correct? Implications for decision support and error reduction. *J Gen Intern Med* 2005;20:334–339.

9. Croskerry P. Achieving quality in clinical decision making: cognitive strategies and detection of bias. *Acad Emerg Med* 2002;9:1184–1204.

10. Goldman L, Kirtane AJ. Triage of patients with acute chest pain and possible cardiac ischemia: the elusive search for diagnostic perfection. *Ann Intern Med* 2003;139:987–995.

ADDITIONAL READINGS

Gladwell M. *Blink: The Power of Thinking Without Thinking.* New York, NY: Little, Brown and Company, 2005.

Graber M. Diagnostic errors in medicine: a case of neglect. *Jt Comm J Qual Saf* 2005;31:106–113.

Groopman J. *How Doctors Think.* Boston, MA: Houghton Mifflin, 2007.

Kahneman D, Slovic P, Tversky A. *Judgment under Uncertainty: Heuristics and Biases.* Cambridge, England: Cambridge University Press, 1987.

Kassirer JP, Kopelman RI. Cognitive errors in diagnosis: instantiation, classification, and consequences. *Am J Med* 1989;86:433–441.

Redelmeier DA. Improving patient care. The cognitive psychology of missed diagnoses. *Ann Intern Med* 2005;142:115–120.

Human Factors and Errors at the Person-Machine Interface[*]

INTRODUCTION

U p until now, we have discussed several paradigm shifts required to improve patient safety. The dominant one, of course, is replacing an environment based on "blame and shame" with one in which safety is viewed as a top priority and systems thinking is effectively employed. Second is an awareness of the impact of culture and relationships on communication and the exchange of information. This chapter will introduce another lens through which to view safety problems: how human factors engineering (HFE) can improve the safety of man-machine interactions and the environment in which healthcare providers work.

To prime ourselves for a discussion of HFE, consider the following scenarios:

- Intensive care unit (ICU) or surgical patients sometimes have their temperature monitored through a probe placed in their Foley catheter. This probe can rapidly become superheated—enough to perforate an organ—in an MRI scanner.

---

[*]This chapter was coauthored by Bryan Haughom.

- Modern multichannel infusion pumps are routinely used in the ICU to administer multiple medications and fluids through a single central line. This often results in a confusing tangle of tubes that cannot be easily differentiated. No surprise, then, that a busy ICU nurse might adjust the dose of the wrong medication.

- Medications are often stored in vials that are far more concentrated than the dose at which they are administered. For example, a vial of phenylephrine contains 10 mg/mL. The usual IV dose administered to patients is 0.1 mg—one-hundredth of the dose in the vial! Inadvertent administration of full strength phenylephrine can cause a stroke.

In each of these examples, significant hazards result from people interacting with products, tools, procedures, and processes in the clinical environment. One could argue that errors in these circumstances could be prevented by more vigilant clinicians or more robust training. However, as we have already learned, it is critical to apply systems thinking to minimize the chances that fallible humans will cause patient harm. In the case of person-machine interfaces, this systems focus leads us to consider issues around device design, the environment, and the care processes that accompany device use. The field of HFE provides the tools to consider these issues.

HUMAN FACTORS ENGINEERING

Human factors engineering is an applied science of systems design that is concerned with the interplay among humans, machines, and their work environments.[1, 2] HFE's goal is to assure that devices, systems, and working environments are designed to minimize the likelihood of error and optimize safety. As one of its central tenets, the field recognizes that humans are fallible and that they often overestimate their abilities and underestimate their limitations. Human factors engineers strive to understand the strengths and weaknesses of human physical and mental abilities and use that information to design safer devices, systems, and environments.

HFE is a hybrid field, mixing various engineering disciplines, design, and cognitive psychology. Its techniques have long been used in the highly complex and risky fields of aviation, electrical power generation, and petroleum refining, but its role in patient safety has only recently been appreciated.[3–5] In applying HFE to healthcare, there has been a particular emphasis on the design and use of devices such as intravenous pumps, catheters, computer software and hardware, and the like.

Devices are a frequent target of HFE techniques. Many medical devices have poorly designed user interfaces, both confusing and clumsy to use.[6,7] In fact, the U.S. Food and Drug Administration (FDA) noted that approximately half of all medical device recalls between 1985 and 1989 stemmed from poor design. FDA officials, along with other human factors experts, now recognize the importance of integrating human factors principles into the design of medical equipment.[6,8,9]

In Chapter 2, we introduced the concept of "forcing functions," design features that prevent the user from taking an action without deliberately considering information relevant to that action. In healthcare, forcing functions have been created to, for example, make it impossible to connect the wrong gas canisters to an anesthetized patient or prevent patients from overdosing themselves while receiving patient-controlled analgesia (PCA). Although forcing functions are the most straightforward application of HFE, it is important to appreciate other healthcare applications—ranging from device design, to aiding in device procurement decisions, to evaluating processes within the care environment. For example, many hospitals are now approaching the challenge of increasing the frequency with which providers clean their hands as, in part, a human factors problem (Chapter 10).[10] While these institutions continue to focus on education and observation, they also ensure that cleaning gel dispensers are easy to use and strategically located throughout the hospital wards. Extending this example, a whole field of patient safety-centered hospital and clinic design has emerged, with some buildings being constructed around human factors principles.[11]

Despite these early success stories, HFE remains conspicuously underused as a patient safety tool, for reasons ranging from the lack of well-defined avenues to report and correct design or process flaws within hospitals to the natural tendency of highly trained caregivers to feel that they can outsmart or work around problems.[5] But they also relate to a failure to recognize the growing complexity of modern care delivery. With the dramatic growth in the volume and complexity of man-machine interactions in the clinical environment, the probability that fallible human workers will make mistakes has escalated, as has the importance of considering HFE approaches to safety issues.

USABILITY TESTING AND HEURISTIC ANALYSIS

One of the key tools in HFE is "usability testing," in which experts observe frontline workers engaging in their task under realistic conditions—either actual patient care or simulated environments that closely replicate actual conditions. Users are observed, videotaped, and asked to "talk through" their thought processes, explaining their actions as well as their difficulties with a given application or device. Engineers then analyze the data in order to fine-tune their design for the users, the chosen tasks, and the work environment.[12]

Software engineers and design firms now see usability testing as an indispensable part of their work, preferring to make modifications at the design stage instead of waiting until errors have become apparent through real world use. Similarly, many equipment manufacturers and a growing number of healthcare organizations now employ individuals with human factors expertise to advise them on equipment purchasing decisions, modify existing equipment to prevent errors, or identify error-prone equipment and environmental situations. These trained individuals instinctively approach errors with a human factors mindset, asking questions about usability and possible human factors solutions before considering solutions involving retraining and incentives, interventions that may seem easier than device or environmental redesign but are generally far less effective.

Usability testing can be a rather involved process, requiring not only human factors experts but extensive investigatory time and cooperation from users. A less resource intensive alternative has emerged in the form of heuristic analysis.[7] The term *heuristics* was first mentioned in Chapter 6 in reference to the cognitive shortcuts that clinicians often take during diagnostic reasoning, shortcuts that can sometimes lead to errors. However, in the context of HFE, heuristics have a different connotation: "rules of thumb" or governing principles for device or system design. In heuristic evaluations, the usability of a particular system or device is assessed by applying established design fundamentals such as visibility of system status, user control and freedom, consistency and standards, flexibility, and efficiency of use[12,13] (Table 7–1).

During a heuristic evaluation, experts navigate the user interface searching for usability issues. In essence, analysts try to put themselves in the shoes of the end user, looking for error-prone functions, capabilities, or designs that might ultimately compromise patient safety. The information gleaned from these analyses becomes feedback to the design teams, who iteratively update and refine the design of prototypes. The ultimate shortcoming of heuristics, however, is that they are only as good as the analyst performing the evaluation. Without putting end users in real-time situations and observing their work, it is difficult to fully unearth problematic design issues. Nevertheless heuristic evaluations can provide valuable information to a design team, or even to a hospital looking to review current devices or systems they may already own or devices they are looking to purchase.[4,7]

TABLE 7–1 **Examples of heuristic principles**	
Visibility of system status	Users should be aware of system status System should provide appropriate feedback as well as appropriate instructions to complete a task
User control and freedom	Users should feel "in control" of a system System should provide clear exits at every step of a task, supply undo as well as redo functions, and avoid irreversible actions
Match between system and world	Language utilized by the system should be that of the end user System should fit within the mental model of the end user
Consistency and standards	User interface and system functions should be consistent
Recognition rather than recall	Memory load should be minimized Systems should take advantage of user's inherent tendency to process information in "chunks" as opposed to by rote memory
Flexibility and efficiency of use	Interfaces should be designed to accommodate customizability
Error recovery and prevention	Systems should be designed to prevent errors before they occur If errors do occur, users should be able to recover from them via reversible actions The system should also provide clear steps detailing how to recover
Help and documentation	Help and documentation should be available to users The language used should be appropriate for the end user, avoid jargon

Reproduced with permission from Ginsburg G. Human factors engineering: a tool for medical device evaluation in hospital procurement decision-making. *J Biomed Inform* 2005;38:213–219; Zhang J, Johnson TR, Patel VL, et al. Using usability heuristics to evaluate patient safety of medical devices. *J Biomed Inform* 2003;36:23–30; Kushniruk AW, Patel VL. Cognitive and usability engineering methods for the evaluation of clinical information systems. *J Biomed Inform* 2004;37:56–76.

Inability to truly stand in for the novice is only one problem that designers and engineers have in anticipating all the safety hazards of complex systems. Don Norman, the author of the best-selling book, *The Design of Everyday Things*,[14] reflected on another real-world human factors issue:

[As an engineer], you focus too much, and don't appreciate that all the individual elements of your work, when combined together, create a system—one that might be far more error-prone than you would have predicted from each of the individual components. For example, the anesthesiologist may review beforehand what is going to be needed. And so he or she picks up the different pieces of equipment that measure the different things, like the effects of the drugs on the patient. Each instrument actually may be designed quite well, and it may even have been rigorously tested. But each instrument works differently. Perhaps each has an alarm that goes off when something's wrong. Sounds good so far. But when you put it together as a system it's a disaster. Each alarm has a different setting, and the appropriate response to one may be incredibly dangerous for another. When things really go wrong, all the alarms are beeping and the resulting cacophony of sounds means nobody can get any work done. Instead of tending to the patient, you're spending all of your time turning off the alarms. So part of the problem is not seeing it as a system, that things have to work in context. And that these items actually should be talking to each other so that they can help the anesthesiologist prioritize the alarms.[15]

The difficulty of anticipating all these interactions and dependencies is yet another powerful argument for usability testing, not only of individual devices but of multiple devices as they interact in real world systems.

In addition to their use in the design and purchase of medical devices such as ventilators, programmable IV pumps, defibrillators, and anesthesia equipment, human factors principles can also be utilized in the design and implementation of advanced information technology systems (Chapter 13). Examples include designing the user interface of an electronic medical record to assure important clinical information is not overlooked, designing bar coding systems to maximize medication safety, and designing computerized provider order entry (CPOE) systems to maximize reliability and patient safety. Human factors techniques can also be used to increase the safety of a working environment, such as by standardizing devices within a hospital to make training easier and increase reliability, carefully designing equipment and processes in a pharmacy to assure pharmacists always dispense the right drug in the correct dose, and optimizing a clinical work environment by providing adequate lighting, eliminating distractions (including excess noise), and ensuring that care providers receive adequate rest.

In the end, usability testing and heuristic analysis can be used together or separately to design safe, effective, and intuitive devices for use in complex clinical care situations. Let's now return to the clinical scenarios outlined at the beginning of the chapter. How could HFE principles be applied to prevent these unsafe conditions? Here are some approaches human factors engineers might consider for each scenario:

- Temperature probes could be designed using materials that do not overheat in a strong magnetic field. Alternatively, probes could be designed to provide a warning if they come in the presence of a strong magnetic field or if they heat beyond physiologic levels.

- Using standard color coding and other techniques, IV lines can be more easily differentiated when nurses are using multichannel infusion pumps.

- Pharmacies can be equipped with high reliability robotic systems that produce bar coded unit-dose medications that can be double-checked using bar coding devices at the bedside before they are administered to the patient.

A case study in the application of HFE to a patient safety problem, adapted from the book *Set Phasers on Stun*,[16] is described in Box 7–1.

BOX 7–1

A CASE STUDY OF FATAL ERROR THAT MIGHT HAVE BEEN PREVENTED BY A HFE APPROACH

HM was a 4-year-old girl with a complex history including birth defects and cardiac problems. She was no stranger to the hospital, to the telemetry unit, or to its nurses. Nurse K carefully attended to her fragile patient, ensuring that each of the six ECG leads were properly placed on HM's small body. As soon as they were all in place, Nurse K gently folded the bed sheet over HM's frail torso, and tucked her into bed. After properly connecting the ECG leads to the patient, the final step was to plug them into the heart monitor, which would allow the nurses to observe HM's heart rhythm at the nursing station down the hall.

After Nurse K lifted the guardrail on the side of the bed, she grabbed the ECG cord and scanned the head of the bed for the connection to the monitor. As was typical in this unit, there were several machines at the bedside—in this case, including an ECG machine and an IV infusion pump. The cord connected to the ECG leads in her hand had a characteristic six-pin connector at the end. It was designed such that it would fit perfectly with its counterpart. She grabbed the cord that was dangling down next to the heart monitor, lined up the two ends and pushed them together. It didn't even cross her mind that the cord she had just connected could potentially be from something other than the ECG machine. After all, she was a seasoned nurse who handled these machines every day, and they all seemed to have different connecting pins.

(Continued)

> ## BOX 7–1 (*Continued*)
>
> Unbeknownst to her she had connected the ECG leads to the IV infusion pump. The cord from the infusion pump matched the size and shape of the six-pin ECG cord reasonably well. The similarity might not have been so dangerous had the infusion pump not been a battery powered portable model. Nurse K had no way to know she had been holding a live electrical wire, with the full electrical current of the IV pump. Connecting the cords delivered a direct shock to the little girl's chest, from which she could not be revived.
>
> Though it may be easy to simply claim that Nurse K should have paid closer attention to the situation, it would be an incomplete analysis. Even if she had been paying attention, would she have committed this fateful error? We may never know. However, looking at this case through a human factors lens reveals a number of potential pitfalls to which Nurse K fell victim. The most glaring is the similarity between the ECG and IV pump cord. Despite the fact that they weren't perfect matches, they matched closely enough that one could connect the two. The most powerful HFE solution might be designing the two connections to have unique colors or shapes—the ECG cord round, and the IV pump cord square, for example. Perhaps the device industry might be willing to subscribe to a set of standards such that all ECG cords have the same color and shape (ditto for pump cords). Another solution might be to have a warning label on the infusion pump's cord, alerting that it can deliver a direct and potentially fatal current.
>
> Even beyond the design of the devices, what other problems may have led this child's death? Could the conditions of the room—the set up, the lighting, the ambient noise, or the nurse's workload played a role in the outcome? Maybe Nurse K wasn't used to seeing these particular device models in the same room. Maybe the demands of her job and the busy environment of a hospital floor were taking their toll. We'll never know for sure. But it is certain that the thoughtful application of HFE principles to this situation would have made it a safer environment.
>
> ---
>
> Reproduced with permission from Casey S., *Set Phasers on Stun: And Other True Tales of Design, Technology, and Human Error, 2nd ed.* Santa Barbara, CA: Aegean Publishing, 1998.

KEY POINTS

- Human factors engineering (HFE) is the applied science of systems design. It is concerned with the interplay of humans, machines, and their work environments.

- Thoughtful application of HFE principles can help prevent errors at the person-machine interface.

- Usability testing and heuristic analysis aim to idenfity error-prone devices or systems before they lead to harm.

- The initial focus of HFE in healthcare was on the design of medical devices. Today it is broader, with efforts to try to create safe environments of care (i.e., designing hospital rooms around safety principles) and to decrease errors associated with poorly designed clinical information systems.

REFERENCES

1. Weinger MB, Pantiskas C, Wiklund M, et al. Incorporating human factors into the design of medical devices. *JAMA* 1998;280:1484.
2. Schneider PJ. Applying human factors in improving medication-use safety. *Am J Health Syst Pharm* 2002;59:1115–1119.
3. Kohn LT, Corrigan JM, Donaldson MD. *To Err is Human—Building a Safer Health System*. Washington, DC: National Academy Press, 1999.
4. Ginsburg G. Human factors engineering: a tool for medical device evaluation in hospital procurement decision-making. *J Biomed Inform* 2005;38:213–219.
5. Wears RL, Perry SJ. Human factors and ergonomics in the emergency department. *Ann Emerg Med* 2002;40:206–212.
6. Lin L, Isla R, Doniz K, et al. Applying human factors to the design of medical equipment: patient-controlled analgesia. *J Clin Monitor Comput* 1998;14:253–263.
7. Zhang J, Johnson TR, Patel VL, et al. Using usability heuristics to evaluate patient safety of medical devices. *J Biomed Inform* 2003;36:23–30.
8. Food and Drug Administration. Human Factors Implications of the new GMP Rule. Overall Requirements of the New Quality System Regulations. Available at: http://www.fda.gov/cdrh/humfac/hufacimp.html.
9. Sawyer D, Aziz KJ, Backinger CL, et al. *Do it by Design: An Introduction to Human Factors in Medical Devices*. US Department of Health and Human Services, Public Health Service, Food and Drug Administration, Center for Devices and Radiological Health, 1996.
10. Gawande A. *Better: A Surgeon's Notes on Performance*. New York, NY: Metropolitan Books, 2007.
11. Facilities Guidelines Institute, AIA Academy of Architecture for Health. *2006 Guidelines for Design and Construction of Health Care Facilities*. Washington, DC: The American Institute of Architects, 2006.
12. Kushniruk AW, Patel VL. Cognitive and usability engineering methods for the evaluation of clinical information systems. *J Biomed Inform* 2004; 37:56–76.
13. Nielsen J. *Usability Engineering*. New York, NY: Academic Press, 1993.

14. Norman DA. *The Design of Everyday Things*. New York, NY: Basic Books, 2002.
15. Norman DA. In conversation with... Donald A. Norman. AHRQ WebM&M (serial online), November 2006. Available at: http://webmm.ahrq.gov/perspective.aspx?perspectiveID = 33.
16. Casey SM. *Set Phasers on Stun: And Other True Tales of Design, Technology, and Human Error*. Santa Barbara, CA: Aegean Publishing Company, 1998.

ADDITIONAL READINGS

Cooper JB, Newbower RS, Long CD, et al. Preventable anesthesia mishaps: a study of human factors. *Anesthesiology* 1978;49:399–406.

France DJ, Throop P, Walczyk B, et al. Does patient-centered design guarantee patient safety? Using human factors engineering to find a balance between provider and patient needs. *J Patient Saf* 2005;1:145–153.

Gosbee J. Human factors engineering and patient safety. *Qual Saf Health Care* 2002;11:352–354.

Gosbee J. Human factors engineering can teach you how to be *surprised* again. AHRQ WebM&M (serial online), November 2006. Available at: http://webmm.ahrq.gov/perspective.aspx?perspectiveID=32.

Tenner E. *Why Things Bite Back: Technology and the Revenge of Unintended Consequences*. New York, NY: A. A. Knopf, 1996.

CHAPTER EIGHT

Transition
and Handoff
Errors

*A*n 83-year-old man with a history of chronic obstructive pulmonary disease (COPD), gastroesophageal reflux disease, and
paroxysmal atrial fibrillation with sick sinus syndrome was
admitted to the cardiology service of a teaching hospital for
initiation of an antiarrhythmic medication and placement of a
permanent pacemaker.

*The patient underwent pacemaker placement via the left subclavian
vein at 2:30 p.m. A routine post-op single view radiograph was
taken and showed no pneumothorax. The patient was sent to the
recovery unit for overnight monitoring. At 5:00 p.m., the patient
stated he was short of breath and requested his COPD inhaler. He
also complained of new left-sided back pain. The nurse found that
his oxygenation had dropped from 95% to 88%. Supplemental oxygen was started and the nurse asked the covering physician to see
the patient. The patient was on the nurse practitioner (NP) non-
housestaff service; however the on-call intern provides coverage for
patients after the NPs leave for the day. The intern, who had never
met the patient before, examined him and found him already feeling
better and with improved oxygenation with the supplemental oxygen. The nurse suggested a stat x-ray be done in light of the recent
surgery. The intern concurred and the portable x-ray was completed
within 30 minutes. About an hour later, the nurse wondered about
the x-ray and asked the covering intern if he had seen it. The intern
stated that he was signing out the x-ray to the night float resident,
who was coming on duty at 8:00 p.m.*

*Meanwhile, the patient continued to feel well except for mild
back pain. The nurse gave him analgesics and continued to*

monitor his heart rate and respirations. At 10:00 p.m., the nurse still hadn't heard anything about the x-ray so she called the night float resident. The night float had been busy with an emergency but promised to look at the x-ray and advise the nurse if there was any problem. Finally at midnight, the nurse signed out to night shift, mentioning the patient's symptoms and noting that the night float had not called with any bad news.

The next morning, the radiologist read the x-ray performed at 6:00 p.m. and notified the NP that it showed a large left pneumothorax. A chest tube was placed at 2:30 p.m. nearly a full day after the x-ray was performed. Luckily, the patient suffered no long-lasting harm from the delay.[1]

SOME BASIC CONCEPTS AND TERMS

Handoff and transitional errors are among the most common and consequential errors in healthcare. Despite this, these errors received little attention until recently, in part because, by their very nature, they tend to fall between the cracks of professional silos. As we have come to recognize the frequency and impact of these errors, we are beginning to learn how to mitigate the harm that often accompanies handoffs.

Healthcare is chock-full of two kinds of transitions and handoffs.[2] The first are patient-related, as a patient moves from place to place within the healthcare system, either within the same building or from one location to another (Table 8–1). The second kind of handoff occurs even when patients are stationary, because there are many handoffs of information that occur between and among providers (Table 8–2). Both kinds of handoffs are fraught with hazards. For example, one study found that 12% of patients experienced preventable adverse events after hospital discharge, most commonly medication errors.[3] Part of the problem is that nearly half of all discharged patients have test results that are pending at discharge, and many (more than half in one study) fall through the cracks.[4] In another study, researchers found that being covered, principally at night, by a different physician was a far better predictor of hospital complications and errors than was the severity of the patient's illness.[5] The same researchers devised a standardized, computerized sign-out form and the error rate—from that particular gap, at least—fell by a factor of 3.[6]

Because patient- and provider-related transitions create the risk of a "voltage drop" in information, one might reasonably ask whether

TABLE 8–1

Examples of patient-related transitions

- Patient referred from primary care provider to subspecialty consultant
- Patient leaves the emergency department to go to the ICU
- Patient leaves the ICU to obtain a computed tomography (CT) scan
- Patient leaves the hospital to go to a skilled nursing facility

healthcare needs to have so many. The answer is probably yes. Research has demonstrated that patients do worse when nurses work shifts longer than 12 hours, and that intensive care unit (ICU) residents make fewer errors when they work shifts averaging 16 hours instead of the traditional 30–36 hours.[7,8] Unfortunately, in a 24-7 hospital, implementing these shift limits automatically generates handoffs (Figure 8–1), such as many of the ones in this case (Figure 8–2). Other handoffs emerge when patients receive appropriately specialized care: although some might wistfully long for the day when the family doctor saw the patient in the office, the emergency room, the hospital, and the operating and delivery room, most patients now prefer the additional expertise, training, and availability of specialists in the sites of care (i.e., emergency department, ICU, and increasingly the hospital), procedure (delivering a baby), or disease (heart attack or stroke). As these specialists become involved in a patient's care, they create transitions and the need for accurate information transfer. So too does a patient's need to escalate the level of care (such as transition from hospital floor to step-down unit) or the economic realities that often necessitate deescalation (hospital to skilled nursing facility).

TABLE 8–2

Examples of provider-related transitions (when patient is stationary)

- Daytime resident signs out to night float resident
- Oncologist's partner covers over a weekend
- Nightshift nurse leaves, morning nurse takes over
- Recovery room nurse goes on break

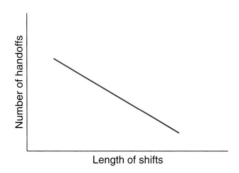

FIGURE 8–1.   The tradeoff between shift length and handoffs.

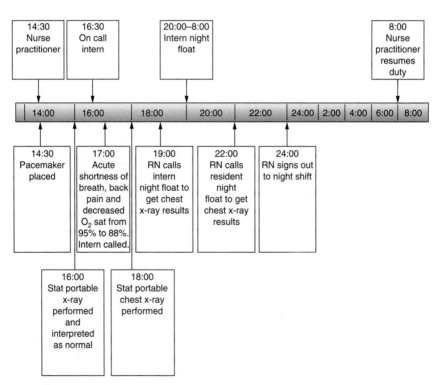

FIGURE 8–2.   Handoffs in this chapter's case. (Reproduced with permission from Vidyarthi AR. Triple handoff. AHRQ WebM&M (serial online), September 2006. Available at: http://www.webmm.ahrq.gov/case.aspx?caseID=134.)

The presence of all these handoffs and transitions makes it critical to consider how information is passed between providers and places. Catalyzed in part by the mandated reduction in consecutive work hours by residents in the United States that began in 2003 (Chapter 16), there has been far more attention paid to handoffs in recent years. In our institution, for example, the number of handoffs by internal medicine residents rose by 40% after duty hours limits were implemented.[9] With this attention has come a deeper understanding of best practices, which have both structural and interpersonal components.

BEST PRACTICES FOR PERSON-TO-PERSON HANDOFFS

Like many other areas of patient safety, the search for best practices in handoffs has led us to examine how other industries and organizations move information around. This search has revealed several elements of effective handoffs: an information system, a predictable and standardized structure, and robust interpersonal communication. In 2006, these requirements were codified in a Joint Commission National Patient Safety Goal (Appendix IV), which requires all healthcare providers to "implement a standardized approach to handoff communications including an opportunity to ask and respond to questions." The Joint Commission's expectations include interactive communications, up-to-date and accurate information, limited interruptions, a process for verification, and an opportunity to review any relevant historical data.

Vidyarthi and colleagues have developed the mnemonic "*ANTICi-pate*" to help structure written sign-outs (Table 8–3). For example, in the above case, listing "Tasks" in the form of "if, then" statements might have decreased the ambiguity. The written sign-out might have included "Check the chest x-ray taken at 6 p.m. If clear, call the nurse. If it shows a pneumothorax, call thoracic surgery for possible chest tube." Contingency plans could have taken the form of "if the patient is short of breath, try an albuterol inhaler (history of COPD), but also consider pneumothorax (patient had recent line placement)."[1]

Written sign-outs can take a variety of forms, but there is an increasing recognition of the advantages of *computerized sign-out systems* over traditional index cards. At the University of California, San Francisco (UCSF) Medical Center, we have developed a computerized sign-out

TABLE 8–3
The mnemonic "ANTICipate," highlighting the elements of a safe and effective handoff

Administrative	Accurate information, such as name and location
New information	A clinical update, including brief history and diagnosis, updated medication and problem list, current baseline status, and recent procedures and significant events
Tasks	The "to do" list, best expressed in "if/then" statements
Illness	The primary provider's assessment of the patient's severity of illness
Contingency plans	Statements that assist in cross-coverage, including things that have and have not worked in the past

Reproduced with permission from Vidyarthi AR. Triple handoff. AHRQ WebM&M (serial online), September 2006. Available at: http://www.webmm.ahrq.gov/case.aspx?caseID=134.

module ("Synopsis"), which resides within the electronic medical record (Figure 8–3). The template standardizes the content of the sign-out and allows multiple providers to see the same data. It also imports certain information from the remainder of the electronic medical record (including administrative information, vital signs, laboratory studies, medication lists, and resuscitation ["code"] status). As one might expect, systems like this improve the quality of sign-outs and decrease the risk of communication-related errors.[6,10]

Computers are an essential part of the answer, but only part. Even in systems that enjoy advanced computerized records, person-to-person communication remains both necessary and potentially error prone. In civil and military aviation, fields that (like healthcare) depend on the accurate transmittal of information, the so-called *phonetic alphabet* is often used during voice communications. In this system, a standardized word substitutes for a single letter (such as *Alpha* for "A," *Bravo* for "B," *Charlie* for "C," and so on), which permits one person to clarify a bit of information, such as the spelling of a name, without wasting time thinking of words that might have a common reference. Using this same system in a hospital, "Oscar Romeo" for operating room (OR) would never be confused with "Echo Romeo" for ER.

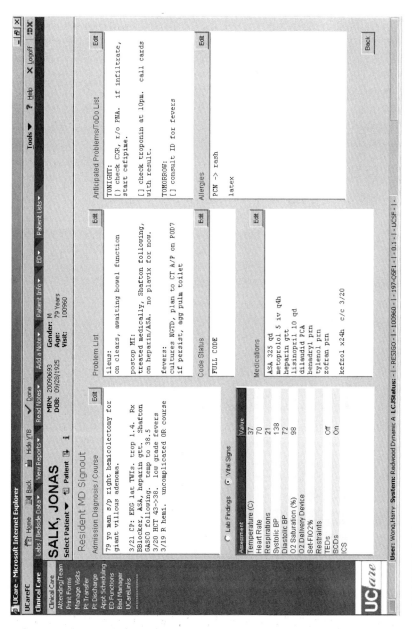

FIGURE 8–3. "Synopsis"—the UCSF Medical Center handoff module embedded in an electronic medical record. Reproduced with permission.

91

Read backs are also commonly used in aviation (and other industries) to prevent improperly received messages. For example, a pilot receiving flight plan clearance over the radio from Air Traffic Control always reads it back. In healthcare, we have long used read-back procedures to verify the identity of blood transfusion recipients, but, remarkably, no tradition of read backs for other transfers of risky information existed until the process was mandated by the Joint Commission in 2004. It is one measure of our inattention to patient safety that a physician would have been far more likely to hear the words, "Let me read your order back to you," when calling her local Chinese takeout restaurant than when she called the nurses' station of virtually any U.S. hospital until very recently.[11] In one study of 822 telephone calls for critical laboratory test results, read backs caught 29 errors (3.5%), some of them quite serious.[12]

BEST PRACTICES FOR SITE-TO-SITE HANDOFFS

Joe Silber (a pseudonym), a 43-year-old mechanic, came to his local ER with chest pain, and was admitted to the hospital to "rule-out MI." Silber's ER physician ordered a chest radiograph in addition to the cardiac enzymes and serial electrocardiograms. Since nobody expected Silber's x-ray to show anything exciting, and since there was no checklist or protocol to remind anyone to check it, it was forgotten as soon as it was taken. Twelve hours later, after all of the heart attack tests proved negative, Silber was discharged. The discharging hospitalist, unaware of the chest x-ray, didn't think to check its results. Meanwhile, the radiologist had reviewed the x-ray and noticed a small lung nodule. He filled out a report for the hospital chart, and sent a version of it to the patient's primary care physician's office, where it was lost.

Two years later, Joe Silber developed a chronic cough and a repeat chest x-ray revealed an obvious lung nodule. The radiologist's report read, "The nodule is markedly enlarged compared to the one seen on the x-ray of October 18, 1999." That was the first Silber's primary physician had heard of the prior x-ray, and it was too late. Eighteen months later, Joe Silber was dead of lung cancer.[11]

In its 2001 report, *Crossing the Quality Chasm: A New Health System for the 21st Century*, the Institute of Medicine analogized the U.S.

healthcare delivery system to a railroad whose tracks change gauge every few miles:

> Health care is composed of a large set of interacting systems—paramedic, emergency, ambulatory, inpatient, and home health care; testing and imaging laboratories; pharmacies; and so forth—that are connected in loosely coupled but intricate networks of individuals, teams, procedures, regulations, communications, equipment, and devices. These systems function within such diverse and diffuse management, accountability, and information structures that the overall term *health system* is today a misnomer.[13]

One potential failure point in all of these interlocking systems is the piece of paper, the basic unit of medical record keeping for centuries. Moving paper across healthcare transitions is inherently risky, as paper can easily get lost. Moreover, several people, separated in place and by function, often need to simultaneously see patient data, and each may create new data and observations that need to be added to the record. Paper is clearly not the ideal media for this.

Many of the handoff techniques discussed earlier can help here as well—including the use of read backs, standard communication protocols, and checklists (such as for hospital discharge) for patients/families (Table 8–4) and providers (Table 8–5). But part of the problem relates to the absence of integration in most of American medicine. Take, for example, hospital discharge—an inherently risky transition. In the United States, the hospital discharging the patient and the physician receiving the patient are usually not part of the same organization (in most cases, the physician is an independent or small group practitioner). Therefore, the physician's office information system, even if it is computerized, will rarely communicate effectively with the hospital's system, and vice versa. This is a formula for a voltage drop...at a most critical time.

Integrated systems of care—in which the same organization owns or runs the doctor's office, the nursing home, and the hospital—have an advantage in this regard over the rest of us. Patients who leave a United States Veteran's Affairs (VA) hospital for a nursing home generally go to a VA-owned facility; the same is true for patients in the huge Kaiser Permanente system and the other large integrated delivery systems such as the National Health Service in the United Kingdom. The reason these handoffs generally go better is partly organizational, partly psychological, and partly informational. Organizationally, when a single system is

TABLE 8−4
A patient/family discharge checklist

You are about to be discharged from the hospital. Please be sure you and/or your family members know the answer to these questions BEFORE you leave:

Do you understand why you were hospitalized, what your diagnosis is, and what treatments you received?

Are there any test results you are still waiting for? Who should you contact for those results?

Has a provider reviewed your medications with you? Do you know which of your home medications to continue, what the current doses are, and which you should stop taking?

Where and when are your follow-up appointments?

What are the warning signs of relapse or medication side effects you should look for?

Who should you contact if you are having difficulties?

Does your primary care physician know you were here and that you are leaving?

Reproduced with permission from Forster A. Discharge fumbles. AHRQ WebM&M (serial online), December 2004. Available at: http://webmm.ahrq.gov/case.aspx?caseID=84.

responsible for care on both sides of a specialty or facility gap, they collaborate on smoothing the transition and bear the consequence of any problems. Psychologically, human beings simply communicate better with colleagues than with strangers. Finally, from an informatics standpoint, large integrated systems tend to devote more resources to constructing, maintaining, and improving the computer systems so critical to communication. And, unlike the rest of the U.S. healthcare system, where the computer systems are likely to be in silos that may not "speak to each other," integrated systems put a premium on "interoperability."

Recognizing that most of the American healthcare system will remain fragmented for the foreseeable future, much of the federal effort to computerize U.S. healthcare is presently focused on creating a set of standards and protocols that will allow for interoperability, even when the computers are from different vendors and are owned by different organizations (Chapter 13). The best analogy is banking's automatic teller machine (ATM) system, in which the interoperability of ATMs allows customers to make transactions away from their own bank, all over the world.

TABLE 8–5
A caregiver discharge checklist

Discharge medications

Review with the patient

Highlight changes from hospital

Specifically inform patient about side effects

Discharge summaries

Dictate in a timely fashion

Include discharge medications (highlight changes from admission)

List outstanding tests and reports that need follow-up

Give copies to all providers involved in the patient's care

Communication with patient/family

Provide patient with medication instructions, follow-up details, and clear
   instructions on warning signs and what to do if things are not going well

Confirm that patient comprehends your instructions

Include a family member in these discussions if possible

Communication with the primary physician

Make telephone contact with primary care physician prior to discharge

Follow-up plans

Discharge clinic

Follow-up phone calls

Appointments or access to primary providers

Reproduced with permission from Forster A. Discharge fumbles. AHRQ WebM&M (serial
online), December 2004. Available at: http://webmm.ahrq.gov/case.aspx?caseID=84.

Recently, concerns have been raised about patient privacy and the unauthorized use of medical information, and these concerns have taken on additional force with the prospect of large, interoperable computer systems containing mountains of often-sensitive patient data. These concerns, partly addressed in the United States by the 2003 Healthcare Insurance Portability and Accountability Act (HIPAA), pose a real barrier to developing a national medical database, or even to moving patient information from clinic to hospital and back out again. While abuses are possible (and there have already been some high profile examples), policymakers will have to balance the desirability of strict control over patient data against the value of linking healthcare systems in an increasingly mobile society.[14] Both individuals and organizations have experimented with having patients carry their own data (in the form of a "smart cards" or even implantable chips) as a way of addressing these privacy concerns.[15] Because these systems seem a bit too unreliable and inflexible (one big challenge is that they will need to be updated after every clinical encounter), the more realistic hope will be for a single set of national (or even international) standards that would combine seamless interoperability with robust safeguards that ensure reasonable degrees of privacy.

KEY POINTS

- Errors at the time of transitions (also known as handoff errors) are among the most common errors in healthcare.

- Handoffs can be site-to-site (e.g., hospital to skilled nursing faculty) or person-to-person (e.g., one physician signing out to another).

- For both kinds of handoffs, the solutions will involve a combination of information systems and standard protocols.

- Handoffs should occur at designated times and without distraction, cover likely scenarios, include "if/then" statements, and utilize read backs and a phonetic alphabet.

- It will be vital to have computer systems that "talk to each other" ("interoperability"); creating these systems will require that we address legitimate concerns about patient privacy.

REFERENCES

1. Vidyarthi AR. Triple handoff. AHRQ WebM&M (serial online), September 2006. Available at: http://www.webmm.ahrq.gov/case.aspx?caseID=134.
2. Cook RI, Render M, Woods DD. Gaps in the continuity of care and progress on patient safety. *BMJ* 2000;320:791–794.

3. Forster AJ, Murff HJ, Peterson JF, et al. The incidence and severity of adverse events affecting patients after discharge from the hospital. *Ann Intern Med* 2003;138:161–167.

4. Roy CL, Poon EG, Karson AS, et al. Patient safety concerns arising from test results that return after hospital discharge. *Ann Intern Med* 2005; 143:121–128.

5. Petersen LA, Brennan TA, O'Neil AC, et al. Does housestaff discontinuity of care increase the risk for preventable adverse events? *Ann Intern Med* 1994;121:866–872.

6. Petersen LA, Orav EJ, Teich JM, et al. Using a computerized sign-out program to improve continuity of inpatient care and prevent adverse events. *Jt Comm J Qual Improv* 1998;24:77–87.

7. Rogers AE, Hwang WT, Scott LD, et al. The working hours of hospital staff nurses and patient safety. *Health Aff (Millwood)* 2004;23:202–212.

8. Landrigan CP, Rothschild JM, Cronin JW, et al. Effect of reducing interns' work hours on serious medical errors in intensive care units. *N Engl J Med* 2004;351:1838–1848.

9. Vidyarthi AR, Arora V, Schnipper JL, et al. Managing discontinuity in academic medical centers: strategies for a safe and effective resident sign-out. *J Hosp Med* 2006;1:257–266.

10. Van Eaton EG, Horvath KD, Lober WB, et al. A randomized, controlled trial evaluating the impact of a computerized rounding and sign-out system on continuity of care and resident work hours. *J Am Coll Surg* 2005;200:538–545.

11. Wachter RM, Shojania KG. *Internal Bleeding: The Truth Behind America's Terrifying Epidemic of Medical Mistakes*. New York, NY: Rugged Land, 2004.

12. Barenfanger J, Sautter RL, Lang DL, et al. Improving patient safety by repeating (read-back) telephone reports of critical information. *Am J Clin Pathol* 2004;121:801–803.

13. *Crossing the Quality Chasm: A New Health System for the 21ˢᵗ Century*. Committee on Quality of Healthcare in America, Institute of Medicine, 2001.

14. Lo B, Dornbrand L, Dubler NN. HIPAA and patient care: the role for professional judgment. *JAMA* 2005;293:1766–1771.

15. Halamka J. Straight from the shoulder. *N Engl J Med* 2005;353:331–333.

ADDITIONAL READINGS

Arora V, Johnson J, Lovinger D, et al. Communication failures in patient sign-out and suggestions for improvement: a critical incident technique. *Qual Saf Health Care* 2005;14:401–407.

Care Transitions Program. Aurora, CO: The Division of Health Care Policy and Research, University of Colorado Health Sciences Center. Available at: http://www.caretransitions.org/.

Coleman EA, Parry C, Chalmers S, et al. The care transitions intervention: results of a randomized controlled trial. *Arch Intern Med* 2006;166: 1822–1828.

Gandhi TK. Fumbled hand-offs: one dropped ball after another. *Ann Intern Med* 2005;142:352–358.

Kripalani S, LeFevre F, Phillips CO, et al. Deficits in communication and information transfer between hospital-based and primary care physicians: implications for patient safety and continuity of care. *JAMA* 2007;297:831–841.

Laxmisan A, Hakimzada F, Sayan OR, et al. The multitasking clinician: decision-making and cognitive demand during and after team handoffs in emergency care. *Int J Med Inform* 2006 [Epub ahead of print].

Patterson ES, Roth EM, Woods DD, et al. Handoff strategies in settings with high consequences for failure: lessons for health care operations. *Int J Qual Health Care* 2004;16:125–132.

CHAPTER NINE

Teamwork and Communication Errors

A *"Code Blue" is called when a patient on a medical-surgical ward is discovered pulseless and not breathing. The code team rushes in and begins CPR. "Does anybody know this patient?" the team leader barks as the team continues its resuscitative efforts. A few moments later, a resident skids into the room, having pulled the patient's chart from the rack in the nurse's station. "This patient is a No Code!" he blurts, and all activity stops. As the Code Blue team members collect their paraphernalia, the patient's young nurse wonders in silence. After all, she received sign-out on this patient a couple of hours ago, and she was told that the patient was a "full code." She thinks briefly about questioning the physician, but reconsiders. One of the doctors must have changed the patient's Code status to Do Not Resuscitate (DNR) and just forgotten to tell me, she decides. Happens all the time. So she keeps her concerns to herself.*

Only later, after someone picks up the chart that the resident brought into the room, does it become clear that he had inadvertently pulled the wrong chart from the chart rack. The young nurse's suspicions were correct—the patient was a full Code. A second Code Blue was called, but the patient could not be resuscitated.[1]

SOME BASIC CONCEPTS AND TERMS

All organizations need structure and hierarchies, lest there be chaos. Armies must have generals, large organizations must have CEOs, and children must have parents. This is not a bad thing, but taken to extremes, these hierarchies can become so rigid that frontline workers withhold critical information from leaders, or only reveal information they believe their leaders want to hear. This state can easily spiral out of control, leaving the leaders without the information they need to improve the system and the workers believing that the leaders are not listening, are not open to dissenting opinions, and are perhaps not even interested.

The psychological distance between a worker and a supervisor is sometimes called an *authority gradient*, and the overall steepness of this gradient is referred to as the *hierarchy* of an organization. Healthcare has traditionally been characterized by steep hierarchies and very large authority gradients, mostly between physicians and the rest of the workers. Errors like those in the Wrong DNR case have alerted us to the cost of this kind of a hierarchy—in which a young nurse could suspect that something was terribly wrong but not feel comfortable raising her concerns in the face of a physician's forceful (but ultimately incorrect) proclamation.

THE ROLE OF TEAMWORK IN HEALTHCARE

Teamwork may have been less important in healthcare 50 years ago. The pace was slower, the technology less overwhelming, the medications less toxic (also less effective), and quality and safety appeared to be under the control of physicians; everyone else played a supporting role. But the last half century has brought a sea change in the provision of medical care, with massively increased complexity (think liver transplant or electrophysiology), huge numbers of new medications and procedures, and overwhelming evidence that the quality of teamwork often determines whether patients receive appropriate care promptly and safely. As examples, the outcomes of trauma care, obstetrical care, care of the patient with an acute myocardial infarction or stroke, and care of the immunocompromised patient are likely to hinge more on the quality of teamwork than the brilliance of the supervising physician.

As we have come to recognize the importance of teamwork to safety and quality, healthcare has looked to the field of aviation for lessons. In the late 1970s and early 1980s, a cluster of deadly airplane crashes occurred in which a steep authority gradient appeared to be an important causative factor. Probably the best known of these tragedies was the 1977 collision of two 747s on the runway at Tenerife in the Canary Islands.

On March 27, 1977, Captain Jacob Van Zantent, a copilot, and a flight engineer sat in the cockpit of their KLM 747 awaiting clearance to take off on a foggy morning in Tenerife. Van Zantent was revered among KLM employees—as director of safety for KLM's fleet, he was known as a superb pilot. In fact, with tragic irony, in each of the KLM's 300 seat back pockets that morning was an article about him, including his picture. The crew of the KLM had spotted a Pan Am 747 on the tarmac earlier that morning, but it was logical to believe that it was out of the way. The fog hung thick, and there was no ground radar in 1977 to signal to the cockpit crew whether the runway was clear—the crew relied on its own eyes, or those of the air traffic controllers.

A transmission came from the air traffic controllers into the KLM cockpit, but it was garbled—although the crew did glean that it had something to do with the Pan Am 747. Months later, a report from the Spanish Secretary of Civil Aviation described what happened next:

> On hearing this, the KLM flight engineer asked: "Is he not clear then?" The [KLM] captain didn't understand him and [the engineer] repeated, "Is he not clear, that Pan American?" The captain replied with an emphatic, "Yes" and, *perhaps, influenced by his great prestige, making it difficult to imagine an error of this magnitude on the part of such an expert pilot,* both the co-pilot and flight engineer made no further objections.[Italics added][2]

A few moments later, Van Zantent pulled the throttle and his KLM jumbo jet thundered down the runway. Emerging from the fog and now accelerating for takeoff, the pilot saw the Pam Am plane sitting squarely in front of him on the runway. Although he managed to get the nose of the KLM over the Pan Am, doing so required such a steep angle of ascent that his tail dragged along the ground … and through the Pan Am's fuselage. Both planes exploded, causing the deaths of 583 people. Thirty years later, the Tenerife accident remains the worst air traffic collision of all time.

Tenerife and other similar accidents taught aviation leaders the risks of a culture in which it was possible for individuals (such as the KLM flight engineer) to suspect that something was wrong, yet not feel comfortable raising these concerns with the leader. Through many years of teamwork and communications training (called Crew Resource Management, see Chapter 15), commercial airline crews have learned to speak up and raise concerns. Importantly, the programs have also taught pilots how to create an environment that makes it possible for those lower on the authority totem pole to raise issues. The result has been a remarkable safety record in commercial aviation over the past 40 years (Figure 9–1), a record that many experts attribute largely to this "culture of safety"—particularly the dampening of the authority gradient.

How well do we do on this in healthcare? In a 2000 study, Sexton asked members of operating room and aviation crews similar questions about culture, teamwork, and hierarchies.[3] As Figure 9–2 shows, although attending surgeons perceive that teamwork in their operating rooms is quite good, the rest of the "team members" disagree, proving that one should never ask the leader about the quality of teamwork! Perhaps more germane to the patient safety question, while virtually all pilots would welcome being questioned by a coworker or subordinate, nearly 50% of surgeons would not (Figure 9–3).

It is important to recognize that the attitudes now held by surgeons were common among pilots in the past, until pilots recognized that such attitudes (and the culture they represented) made crashes far more likely. As we consider strategies to improve teamwork and dampen down hierarchies in healthcare, it is also worth noting that pilots did not automatically jump for joy at the prospects of teamwork training when it was first introduced in the early 1980s (in fact, many pilots derisively referred to crew resource management training as "charm school"). Yet today it is difficult to find a pilot, or anyone else in commercial aviation, who does not believe that crew resource management and other techniques to improve safety culture and diminish authority gradients have markedly enhanced airline safety. The adaptation of these types of training programs to healthcare is further explored in Chapter 15.

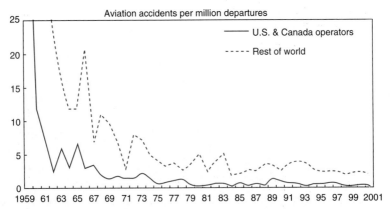

FIGURE 9–1. Commercial aviation's remarkable safety record.

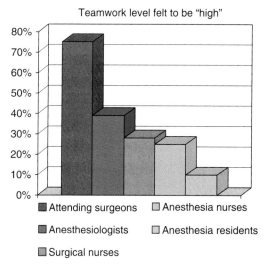

FIGURE 9-2. Percent of providers characterizing teamwork in the OR as "high." (Reproduced with permission from Sexton JB, Thomas EJ, Helmreich RL. Error, stress, and teamwork in medicine and aviation: cross sectional surveys. *BMJ* 2000;320:745-749.)

Finally, as we consider strategies to improve teamwork and dampen hierarchies in healthcare, we would do well to appreciate the complexity of this undertaking and the limitations of the aviation analogy. Changing the cockpit environment to prevent the next Tenerife involved improving teamwork between two or three individuals—captain, first officer, perhaps

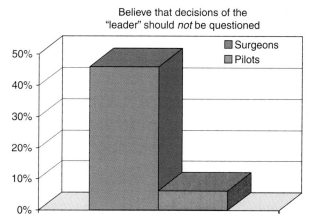

FIGURE 9-3. Percent of pilots and surgeons who would not welcome being questioned by a subordinate. (Reproduced with permission from Sexton JB, Thomas EJ, Helmreich RL. Error, stress, and teamwork in medicine and aviation: cross sectional surveys. *BMJ* 2000;320:745-749.)

flight engineer—who share similar training, expertise, social status, income, and confidence. In a busy operating room, it may be the high school-educated clerk or young nursing assistant who harbors a crucial concern that needs to be transmitted to the senior surgeon. It is important to recognize that transforming *this* culture is far more challenging than changing the culture of the cockpit, and that we are just beginning to learn how to do this effectively in healthcare.

FIXED VERSUS FLUID TEAMS

Some in healthcare point to our fluid teams—the fact that a surgeon is likely to work with a different set of nurses, technicians, and perfusionists every day—as an additional obstacle to improving teamwork. Many do not realize that commercial aviation has precisely the same problem: when you fly a commercial airline, the norm is that your pilot and copilot have never flown together previously. Because fluid teams are so common, it is critical to develop strategies and protocols that do not rely on individuals having worked together to ensure safety. In fact, some observers of both healthcare and aviation have remarked that fixed teams (in which the same group of people work together repetitively) may be *more* dangerous, because they are more likely to get sloppy, make incorrect assumptions, regenerate fixed hierarchies, and suffer from "groupthink."[4]

TEAMWORK AND COMMUNICATION STRATEGIES

Data from the Joint Commission's sentinel event program has demonstrated that communication problems are the most common root cause of serious medical errors (Figure 9–4). Well-functioning teams employ a number of strategies (emphasized in Crew Resource Management training programs) to improve communication and teamwork. The first set of strategies focuses on ways to dampen authority gradients. These efforts can include very simple techniques, such as having the leader introduce him or herself, learn the names of the other workers, admit his or her limitations, and explicitly welcome input from all the members of the team. These techniques can be incorporated into the surgical "time out" described in Chapter 5. But they shouldn't be limited to the presurgical or

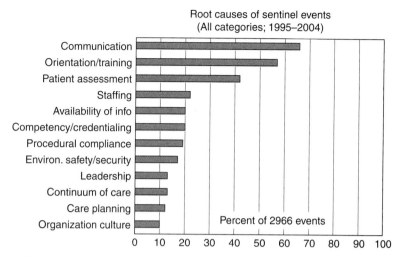

FIGURE 9–4. Frequency of communication problems among Joint Commission sentinel events. Reproduced with permission from The Joint Commission.

procedural hiatus: a medicine attending might employ them on the first day of his or her ward rotation, as might an obstetrician beginning a shift on the labor and delivery floor. For example, a surgeon might introduce himself (and have everyone else do the same) to all the members of his operating room crew, and then say, "You know, there will be times when I miss something, or when I'm going in the wrong direction in the middle of a complicated case. I really depend on all of you to be my eyes and ears. If you see anything that you're not comfortable with—anything—including things that I'm doing, I really want you to bring them up. Together, we can be far safer than any of us can be individually."

There are also powerful opportunities to improve team performance after a procedure or a clinical encounter is over. Known in the military and aviation as a *debriefing*, this involves all team members taking a moment at the end of the procedure and explicitly, in a blame-free way, discussing what went wrong and right.[5] The lessons from these debriefings are often invaluable, and just as importantly, the sessions reinforce the value of team behaviors, the critical importance of speaking up, and the fact that everyone—even the leader—is fallible.

It is one thing to tell nurses, clerks, or medical students to speak up, and another to arm them with tools to do so productively. Many nurses recall having tried to raise concerns with physicians, only to be rebuffed. To improve these exchanges, a number of techniques have been promoted, all designed to ensure that important messages are heard and acted upon. Two of these are SBAR and CUS words.

SBAR stands for "Situation, Background, Assessment, and Recommendations." In most training programs, the focus of SBAR training is on nurses, with SBAR being a way to structure their communication with physicians to capture the latter's attention and generate the appropriate action. The need for SBAR training grew from the recognition that many nurses have been schooled and socialized to report in stories, while physicians have been trained to think and process information in bullet points.[6] For example, a traditional nursing assessment of a postoperative patient with new chest pain might be:

> Hi, doctor. Mr. Chow is having some chest pain. He was walking around the floor earlier, and he ate a good dinner. I don't really know what is going on, but I'm getting an electrocardiogram. He was a little sweaty when he had his pain, but I gave him the rest of his medicines, including his insulin and his antibiotic. He had surgery earlier today, and he's on a PCA pump right now.

After SBAR training, the same nurse might call the physician and say:

> This is Grace Jones. I'm a nurse on 7 North and I'm seeing your patient Edward Chow. He developed 8 out of 10 chest pain about 5 minutes ago, associated with shortness of breath, diaphoresis, and some palpitations (*Situation*). He is a 68-year-old man with no prior history of cardiac disease who had an uncomplicated abdominal-peritoneal resection yesterday (*Background*). I am obtaining an electrocardiogram, and my concern is that he might be having cardiac ischemia or a pulmonary embolism (*Assessment*). I'm giving him a nitroglycerin and would really appreciate it if you could be here in the next five minutes (*Recommendation*).

Another technique to improve communication is the use of *CUS words*. These involve escalating levels of concern, again usually on the part of a nurse (but they would be equally applicable to many other workers: medical students, respiratory therapists, pharmacists—anyone lower on a hierarchy who needs to get the attention of someone higher up). In escalating order, it begins with the use of the words, "I'm *concerned* about …," then "I'm *uncomfortable* …" and finally, "This is a *safety* issue!" It is important to teach those who might be receiving such messages (usually physicians) to appreciate their meaning and respond appropriately, and those who might use CUS words to avoid overusing them, to ensure that they have the intended impact.

Finally, strong teams depend on members—individually and collectively—responding appropriately to crises, particularly when the "fog of war" sets in. The concept of *situational awareness* refers to the degree to which one's perception of a situation matches reality.[7–9] Failure to maintain situational awareness during a crisis can result in various problems that compound the crisis. For instance, during a resuscitation, an individual or entire team may focus on a particular task (such as a difficult central-line insertion or administering a particular medication), while neglecting to address immediately life-threatening problems such as respiratory failure or a pulseless rhythm. In this context, maintaining situational awareness might be seen as equivalent to keeping the "big picture" in mind. Or, to cite one of the famous "Laws of the House of God" (the influential 1979 satire of the world of medical training), "at a cardiac arrest, the first procedure is to take your own pulse."[10]

KEY POINTS

- The provision of high quality, safe healthcare is increasingly a team sport.
- Well-functioning teams are characterized by appropriate authority gradients and hierarchies that don't stifle the free flow of information.
- Healthcare has looked to the field of aviation for guidance regarding how best to dampen down hierarchies; the specific training model in aviation (presently being adapted to healthcare) is known as Crew Resource Management.
- As long as effective teamwork and communication strategies are employed, the presence of fluid (rather than fixed) teams should not be a safety hazard.
- High functioning teams use strategies such as effective introductions and debriefings.
- Strategies to improve communications, particularly up the authority gradient, include the use of SBAR and CUS words.
- Strong teams manage to maintain "situational awareness" (focusing on the big picture) even during crises.

REFERENCES

1. Wachter RM, Shojania KG. *Internal Bleeding: The Truth Behind America's Terrifying Epidemic of Medical Mistakes.* New York, NY: Rugged Land, 2004.
2. Secretary of Aviation (Spain) Report on Tenerife Crash. Aircraft Accident Digest (ICAO Circular 153-AN/56), 1978, pp. 22–68.
3. Sexton JB, Thomas EJ, Helmreich RL. Error, stress, and teamwork in medicine and aviation: cross sectional surveys. *BMJ* 2000;320:745–749.
4. In conversation with . . . Jack Barker. AHRQ WebM&M (serial online), January 2006. Available at: http://webmm.ahrq.gov/perspective.aspx?perspectiveID=17.
5. Makary MA, Holzmueller CG, Sexton JB, et al. Operating room debriefings. *Jt Comm J Qual Patient Saf* 2006;32:407–410, 357.
6. Haig KM, Sutton S, Whittington J. SBAR: a shared mental model for improving communication between clinicians. *Jt Comm J Qual Patient Saf* 2006;32:167–175.
7. Weick KE. The collapse of sensemaking in organizations: the Mann Gulch disaster. *Adm Sci Q* 1993;38:628–652.
8. Weick KE, Sutcliffe KM. *Managing the Unexpected: Assuring High Performance in an Age of Complexity.* San Francisco, CA: Jossey-Bass, 2001.
9. Berwick DM. *Escape Fire: Lessons for the Future of Health Care.* New York, NY: The Commonwealth Fund, 2002.
10. Shem S. *The House of God.* New York, NY: Putnam, 1979.

ADDITIONAL READINGS

Connor M, Ponte PR, Conway J. Multidisciplinary approaches to reducing error and risk in a patient care setting. *Crit Care Nurs Clin North Am* 2002;14:359–367.

Donaldson L. *An Organisation with a Memory: Report of an Expert Group on Learning from Adverse Events in the NHS Chaired by the Chief Medical Officer.* London: The Stationery Office, 2000.

Helmreich RL. On error management: lessons from aviation. *BMJ* 2000; 320:781–785.

Leape LL. Error in medicine. *JAMA* 1994;272:1851–1857.

Sachs BP. A 38-year-old woman with fetal loss and hysterectomy. *JAMA* 2005;294:833–840.

CHAPTER TEN

Nosocomial Infections

GENERAL CONCEPTS AND EPIDEMIOLOGY

To this day, debate continues as to whether an infection caused by failure to adhere to infection control "best practices" (such as properly cleaning one's hands before patient contact) should be classified as a medical error. Before the patient safety movement began, preventing hospital-acquired infections was seen as the job of the hospital epidemiologist and other infection control staff, who tried (often unsuccessfully) to engage clinicians in prevention efforts. Branding healthcare-associated infections as a patient safety problem (which rendered failure to engage in appropriate infection control practices a medical error) has elevated the importance of these infections and propelled prevention into the mainstream. Some have even proposed that certain nosocomial infections be considered sentinel events, each one generating a root cause analysis (Chapter 14).

Gratifyingly, evidence is accumulating that healthcare organizations can markedly decrease the frequency of nosocomial infections. Some hospitals, having religiously implemented a variety of prevention strategies, are reporting months, even years, between previously commonplace infections such as ventilator-associated pneumonias (VAP) and central-line-associated bloodstream infections (Figure 10–1). If, in fact, healthcare-associated infections resulting from failure to adhere to best practices *are* medical errors (and I believe that it is reasonable to consider them as such), then these errors may well be the most common and lethal ones in healthcare.

For many nosocomial infections (and other complications of healthcare, see Chapter 11), a variety of processes or structural changes appear to be correlated with improvement. In the past, infection control experts and regulators emphasized increasing the rate of adhering to individual prevention elements—for example, if there were five strategies thought to be effective

109

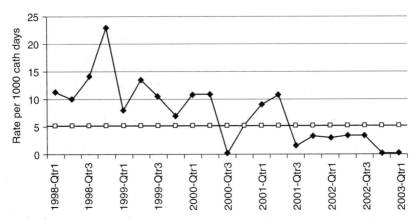

FIGURE 10–1. Marked decrease in catheter-related bloodstream infections after implementation of safety practices at Johns Hopkins Hospital. (Reproduced with permission from Berenholtz SM, Pronovost PJ, Lipsett PA, et al. Eliminating catheter-related bloodstream infections in the intensive care unit. *Crit Care Med* 2004;32:2014–2020.)

in preventing a certain type of infection, a hospital would get "credit" for achieving 100% adherence on one of the five elements, 80% on another, and 50% on the other three. The Institute for Healthcare Improvement (IHI) has promoted the "bundle" approach, emphasizing that the chances of preventing complications seem to be improved when there is complete adherence to a "bundle" of preventive strategies.[1] Under this model, institutions receive credit for their quality and safety efforts only for above-threshold adherence (i.e., >80%) on *all* of the preventive strategies, not just some. The theory behind this approach is that not only does better adherence to the individual elements increase the chances of prevention, but that institutions achieving high all-or-none rates tend to accomplish this by re-engineering the entire clinical process of care. Changes borne of this kind of re-engineering may be more durable than those that result from a short-term project or cheerleading. This theory, though conceptually attractive and useful as a motivational tool, has not been empirically validated.

It is beyond the scope of this book to cover all aspects of healthcare-acquired infections in great detail; the interested reader is referred to other key references.[2,3] Instead, this chapter will highlight some of the patient safety principles involved in preventing healthcare-acquired infections, and end with a discussion of what the patient safety movement can learn from the more established field of infection control.

SURGICAL SITE INFECTIONS

Surgical site infections are among the most common adverse events in hospitalized patients,[4] and result in higher mortality, readmission rates, and costs. Approximately 1 in 30 "clean" surgeries will be complicated by a surgical site infection; the rate is significantly higher for "dirty" (i.e., after trauma), emergency, or prolonged surgeries, and for patients with medical comorbidities. A number of preventive strategies have been developed that appear to result in fewer surgical site infections. The IHI chose four of them for its "5 Million Lives" campaign: appropriate use of prophylactic antibiotics (giving guideline-endorsed antibiotics within an hour of the incision, and stopping it/them within 24 hours after surgery); use of clippers (rather than razors) for hair removal prior to surgery; maintenance of relatively tight glucose control in the postoperative period (best demonstrated to be effective in the surgical intensive care unit [ICU])[5]; and maintenance of postoperative normothermia.[6]

VENTILATOR-ASSOCIATED PNEUMONIA

Ventilator-associated pneumonia is the leading cause of death among hospital-acquired infections, with far more cases of VAP than of nosocomial urinary tract infections, line infections, or surgical site infections.[7] About 15% of patients receiving mechanical ventilation, particularly for long periods, will develop VAP, resulting in prolonged mechanical ventilation and longer hospital stays. Ventilated patients who develop VAP have a significantly higher mortality rate (46%) than those who don't (32%).

We now know that many cases of VAP can be prevented by strict adherence to a variety of preventive strategies. The first is elevation of the head of the bed to semirecumbent (at least 30 degrees) position, which in one trial resulted in an 18% decrease in VAP cases.[8] Head-of-bed (HOB) elevation decreases the risk of microaspiration of gastrointestinal tract and upper respiratory tract secretions into the lungs, which can serve as a nidus for infection. Although this intervention might seem like a relatively simple undertaking, experience has demonstrated that it can be a challenge, usually because of changes in the patient's position.[9] Several tactics have been recommended to increase adherence with HOB elevation, including enlisting the support of respiratory therapists and family members, and placing a visual cue (such as a line on the wall) to help identify whether the bed is in the correct position.

A second effective strategy is daily interruption of sedation for ventilated patients.[10] Under one popular protocol, patients' sedative infusions are stopped each day, allowing patients to "lighten" to the point that they can answer simple questions. This strategy, coupled with a program of systematic assessment (usually by trained respiratory therapists) regarding a patient's suitability for weaning, results in shorter duration of mechanical ventilation, presumably lowering the risk of VAP.[11]

Several other strategies have been included in various "VAP Bundles." The IHI's bundle includes, in addition to the two strategies above, use of prophylaxis for stress gastritis with an H_2 blocker or proton pump inhibitor. Although such prophylaxis is generally recommended in ventilated patients, there is no evidence that it will prevent VAP. The IHI also recommends deep vein thrombosis (DVT) prophylaxis, another appropriate strategy for ventilated patients (see Chapter 11) but one that has not been associated with lower rates of VAP. Finally, a systematic review found that the strategy of continuous drainage of subglottic secretions can lower VAP rates, but the procedure is technically difficult and few institutions utilize it.[12]

The broader topic of hospital-acquired pneumonia will not be covered here. Interested readers are referred to several recent reviews.[13,14]

CATHETER-RELATED BLOODSTREAM INFECTIONS

As catheter access to the central circulation has become ubiquitous in healthcare (to provide long-term antibiotics, nutrition, vasoactive medications, or blood sampling), so too have infectious complications of these lines. The vast majority of catheter-related bloodstream infections (CR-BSI) are associated with central venous catheters (CVCs).[15] Patients in ICUs, nearly half of whom have CVCs, are particularly vulnerable; some estimates put the annual mortality rate from central-line infections at more than 20,000 in the United States alone.[16-18] The IHI-endorsed bundle to prevent central-line infections includes five practices (Table 10–1). Berenholtz has demonstrated that high rates of adherence to these practices (plus another: avoiding the femoral site of catheterization) led to a near-zero rate of CR-BSI in the ICUs at Johns Hopkins Hospital (Figure 10–1). Widespread implementation

---

TABLE 10-1

Elements of the IHI's "bundle" to prevent central-line infections*

---

1. Hand hygiene
2. Maximal barrier precautions
3. Chlorhexidine skin antisepsis
4. Optimal catheter site selection, with subclavian vein as the preferred site for nontunneled catheters
5. Daily review of line necessity, with prompt removal of unnecessary lines

---

*Others, including the group at Johns Hopkins, add avoiding the femoral site of catheterization to the list.

of these practices (accompanied by efforts to improve safety culture) in 100 ICUs in Michigan led to a breathtaking 66% reduction in CR-BSIs over 18 months.[19]

Each of these practices can be facilitated by strong leadership, teamwork, communication (Chapter 15), and an appreciation of human factors (Chapter 7). For example, institutions that have made major gains in hand hygiene often empower nurses (and patients or families; Chapter 21) to question those entering patient rooms about whether they've cleaned their hands, make alcohol-based hand gel dispensers available in conveniently located spots throughout the hospital, and utilize checklists to guide central-line insertions.[20] Similarly, the use of maximal sterile barrier precautions prior to line insertion, which has been strongly associated with lower infection rates,[21] can be facilitated by the use of a dedicated cart containing all the necessary equipment. Importantly, although removal of central lines at the earliest possible date is a key preventive strategy (and should be encouraged by a daily team discussion of the risks versus benefits of continued central access), line replacement (either by a new line at a fresh site or at the same site over a guidewire) does not result in fewer catheter-related infections.[22]

HEALTHCARE-ASSOCIATED URINARY TRACT INFECTIONS

Urinary tract infections are the most common hospital-acquired infections, accounting for about 40% of such infections in the United States. The vast majority are associated with indwelling urinary catheters—risk factors include the duration of catheterization, patient age, and history of malignancy.[23] Although more common than nosocomial pneumonia and catheter-related bloodstream infection, urinary tract infections are less often fatal, and thus have received less attention in the patient safety and infection control literatures.

The strategies for preventing urinary tract infections are similar to those used to prevent central-line infections. Specifically, in patients with indwelling catheters, maintaining a closed drainage system, providing appropriate catheter care, and removing the catheter as quickly as possible have been shown to be beneficial. Saint has demonstrated that nearly one-third of hospital doctors are unaware that their patient has a Foley catheter,[24] and recommends automatic stop orders (after 2 days) or written or computerized provider reminders to ensure that catheters are removed when they are no longer needed.[25,26] In addition to these measures, the use of silver alloy-coated urinary catheters has been associated with fewer infections and is cost-effective for patients who require prolonged catheterization.[27] In men, condom catheters are safer than indwelling catheters.[28]

WHAT CAN PATIENT SAFETY LEARN FROM THE APPROACH TO HOSPITAL-ACQUIRED INFECTIONS?

As a relatively new field, patient safety has largely looked outside of healthcare for lessons—to fields such as commercial aviation, clinical psychology, informatics, and engineering (Chapter 1). However, the patient safety movement can also learn from the much older fields of infection control and hospital epidemiology. Julie Gerberding, Director of the U.S. Centers for Disease Control and Prevention, made this point well in 2002:

> Precise and valid definitions of infection-related adverse events, standardized methods for detecting and reporting events, confidentiality protections, appropriate rate adjustments for institutional and case-mix differences, and evidence-based intervention programs come to mind. Perhaps most important, reliance on skilled professionals to promote ongoing improvements in care has contributed to the 30-year track record of success in infection prevention and control.

> Analogously, in approaching patient safety, standard definitions should be used as much as possible when discussing adverse

events and preventability. Health care organizations should be encouraged to pool data on adverse events in a central repository to permit benchmarking, and such data should be appropriately adjusted and reported. Finally, institutions should consider hiring dedicated, trained patient safety officers (comparable to infection control practitioners). . . .[29]

KEY POINTS

- Recently, infection control activities have been characterized by many as a subset of patient safety, implying that many healthcare-associated infections are caused by medical errors (failure to adhere to evidence-based prevention strategies).

- Many surgical site infections can be prevented by appropriate use of prophylactic antibiotics, clipping rather than shaving the surgical site, and tight postoperative glucose control.

- Many cases of VAP can be prevented by elevating the head of the bed and by strategies designed to minimize the duration of mechanical ventilation (particularly daily interruption of sedation).

- Many CR-BSI and healthcare-acquired urinary tract infections can be prevented by rigorous hand hygiene, strict infection control procedures at the time of insertion, and removal of the foreign bodies at the earliest possible time.

- The new field of patient safety can learn much from the older fields of hospital epidemiology and infection control—particularly, the use of standardized definitions, the importance of data collection and analysis, and the key role of professionals to monitor safety problems and implement safe practices.

REFERENCES

1. Nolan T, Berwick DM. All-or-none measurement raises the bar on performance. *JAMA* 2006;295:1168–1170.
2. Mayhall G. *Hospital Epidemiology and Infection Control*, 3rd ed. Philadelphia, PA: Lippincott Williams and Wilkins, 2004.

3. Wenzel RP. *Prevention and Control of Nosocomial Infections*, 4th ed. Philadelphia, PA: Lippincott Williams and Wilkins, 2002.

4. Brennan TA, Leape LL, Laird NM, et al. Incidence of adverse events and negligence in hospitalized patients. Results of the Harvard Medical Practice Study I. *N Engl J Med* 1991;324:370–376.

5. Van den Berghe G, Wouters P, Weekers F, et al. Intensive insulin therapy in the critically ill patients. *N Engl J Med* 2001;345:1359–1367.

6. Melling AC, Ali B, Scott EM, et al. Effects of preoperative warming on the incidence of wound infection after clean surgery: a randomised controlled trial. *Lancet* 2001;358:876–880.

7. Ibrahim EH, Tracy L, Hill C, et al. The occurrence of ventilator-associated pneumonia in a community hospital: risk factors and clinical outcomes. *Chest* 2001;120:555–561.

8. Drakulovic MB, Torres A, Bauer TT, et al. Supine body position as a risk factor for nosocomial pneumonia in mechanically ventilated patients: a randomized trial. *Lancet* 1999;354:1851–1858.

9. van Nieuwenhoven CA, Vandenbroucke-Grauls C, van Tiel FH, et al. Feasibility and effects of the semirecumbent position to prevent ventilator-associated pneumonia: a randomized study. *Crit Care Med* 2006;34: 396–402.

10. Kress JP, Pohlman AS, O'Connor MF, et al. Daily interruption of sedative infusions in critically ill patients undergoing mechanical ventilation. *N Engl J Med* 2000;342:1471–1477.

11. Esteban A, Frutos F, Tobin MJ, et al. A comparison of four methods of weaning patients from mechanical ventilation. Spanish Lung Failure Collaborative Group. *N Engl J Med* 1995;332:345–350.

12. Dezfulian C, Shojania K, Collard HR, et al. Subglottic secretion drainage for preventing ventilator-associated pneumonia: a meta-analysis. *Am J Med* 2005;118:11–18.

13. Hasan R, Babar SL. Nosocomial and ventilator-associated pneumonias: developing country perspective. *Curr Opin Pulm Med* 2002;8:188–194.

14. Flanders SA, Collard HR, Saint S. Nosocomial pneumonia: state of the evidence. *Am J Infect Control* 2006;34:84–93.

15. Mermel LA. Prevention of intravascular catheter-related infections. *Ann Intern Med* 2000;132:391–402.

16. Pittet D, Tarara D, Wenzel RP. Nosocomial bloodstream infection in critically ill patients. Excess length of stay, extra costs, and attributable mortality. *JAMA* 1994;271:1598–1601.

17. Saint S. Prevention of intravascular catheter-associated infection. In: Shojania KG, Duncan BW, McDonald KM, et al., eds., *Making Health Care Safer: A Critical Analysis of Patient Safety Practices*. Evidence Report/Technology Assessment No. 43, AHRQ Publication No. 01-E058. Rockville, MD: Agency for Healthcare Research and Quality, 2001.

18. Berenholtz SM, Pronovost PJ, Lipsett PA, et al. Eliminating catheter-related bloodstream infections in the intensive care unit. *Crit Care Med* 2004;32: 2014–2020.

19. Pronovost P, Needham D, Berenholtz S, et al. An intervention to decrease catheter-related bloodstream infections in the ICU. *N Engl J Med* 2006; 355:2725–2732.

20. Gawande A. *Better: A Surgeon's Notes on Performance.* New York, NY: Metropolitan Books, 2007.

21. Raad II, Hohn DC, Gilbreath BJ, et al. Prevention of central venous catheter-related infections by using maximal sterile barrier precautions during insertion. *Infect Control Hosp Epidemiol* 1994;15(4 Pt 1):231–238.

22. Cook D, Randolph A, Kernerman P, et al. Central venous catheter replacement strategies: a systematic review of the literature. *Crit Care Med* 1997;25:1417–1424.

23. Nicolle LE. Catheter-related urinary tract infection. *Drugs Aging* 2005; 22:627–639.

24. Saint S, Wiese J, Amory JK, et al. Are physicians aware of which of their patients have indwelling urinary catheters? *Am J Med* 2000;109: 476–480.

25. Saint S, Lipsky BA, Goold SD. Indwelling urinary catheters: a one-point restraint? *Ann Intern Med* 2002;137:125–127.

26. Saint S, Kaufman SR, Thompson M, et al. A reminder reduces urinary catheterization in hospitalized patients. *Jt Comm J Qual Patient Saf* 2005; 31:455–462.

27. Saint S, Veenstra DL, Sullivan SD, et al. The potential clinical and economic benefits of silver alloy urinary catheters in preventing urinary tract infection. *Arch Intern Med* 2000;160:2670–2675.

28. Saint S, Kaufman SR, Rogers MA, et al. Condom versus indwelling urinary catheters: a randomized trial. *J Am Geriatr Soc* 2006;54:1055–1061.

29. Gerberding JL. Hospital-onset infections: a patient safety issue. *Ann Intern Med* 2002;137:665–670.

ADDITIONAL READINGS

Collard HR, Saint S, Matthay MA. Prevention of ventilator-associated pneumonia: an evidence-based systematic review. *Ann Intern Med* 2003;138:494–501.

Hugonnet S, Chevrolet JC, Pittet D. The effect of workload on infection risk in critically ill patients. *Crit Care Med* 2007;35:76–81.

Johnson JR, Kuskowski MA, Wilt TJ. Systematic review: antimicrobial urinary catheters to prevent catheter-associated urinary tract infection in hospitalized patients. *Ann Intern Med* 2006;144:116–126.

Pittet D, Donaldson L. Challenging the world: patient safety and health care-associated infection. *Int J Qual Health Care* 2006;18:4–8.

Shojania KG, Duncan BW, McDonald KM, et al., eds. *Making Health Care Safer: A Critical Analysis of Patient Safety Practices.* Evidence Report/Technology Assessment No. 43, AHRQ Publication No. 01-E058, 2001.

Stelfox HT, Bates DW, Redelmeier DA. Safety of patients isolated for infection control. *JAMA* 2003;290:1899–1905.

CHAPTER ELEVEN

Other Complications of Healthcare

GENERAL CONCEPTS

As with nosocomial infections (Chapter 10), the patient safety movement has broadened the concept of "medical error" to include such outcomes as patient falls, pressure ulcers, and venous thromboembolism (VTE) in the hospitalized patient. Like infection control, the rationale to "lump" rather than "split" is that the strategies to prevent these complications of medical care are similar to those used to prevent other errors. Moreover, as a practical matter, inclusion of these complications under the broad umbrella of patient safety has increased their visibility and the resources available to combat them. This chapter will highlight a few key nosocomial complications and the strategies that can help prevent them.

VENOUS THROMBOEMBOLISM PROPHYLAXIS

Hospitalized or institutionalized patients often have conditions that place them at high risk for VTE, including inactivity, comorbid diseases that increase their risk for clotting (e.g., cancer, nephrotic syndrome, heart failure), and indwelling catheters. Moreover, because such patients often have limited cardiopulmonary reserve, a pulmonary embolism (PE) can be quite consequential, even fatal. In fact, autopsy studies have shown approximately half of patients who die in hospitals will have had a PE, with most of these cases unrecognized antemortem.[1]

The risk of VTE in a hospitalized patient is hard to determine with certainty, because it varies widely depending on the ascertainment method.

Studies relying on clinical diagnosis have found rates of 20% for deep venous thrombosis and 1–2% for PE after major surgical procedures in the absence of prophylaxis. Rates after certain orthopedic procedures are even higher. Studies using more aggressive observational methods (i.e., Doppler ultrasounds on every postoperative patient) have found much higher rates. It is not known how many of these asymptomatic clots would have caused clinical problems, but surely some would have.

A detailed review of strategies to prevent VTE is beyond the scope of this chapter; the interested reader is referred to a number of excellent reviews, particularly the regularly updated guidelines published by the American College of Chest Physicians.[2] Instead, in keeping with the patient safety focus on systems, recent emphasis has been on creating systems that ensure that appropriate, evidence-based prophylaxis is given to every eligible patient. Given the complexity of the VTE prophylaxis decision (which varies by patient group and clinical situation, and changes rapidly with new research and pharmacologic agents), it seems unlikely that physician education, the traditional approach, is the best strategy to ensure that research is translated into practice. Rather, the emphasis should be on developing standardized protocols, through order sets and similar mechanisms and, when possible, building these protocols into computerized decision support systems (Chapter 13). In one study of 2500 hospitalized patients, half the patients received standard care, while the other half's physicians received a computerized notice of their patient's risk status for thromboembolism. The latter group was required to acknowledge the notice and then explicitly choose to withhold prophylaxis or order it (graduated compression stockings, pneumatic boots, unfractionated or low molecular weight heparin, or warfarin). Physicians receiving the alerts were far more likely to order appropriate prophylaxis, and the rates of clinically diagnosed deep venous thrombosis or PE fell by 41%.[3] In a comprehensive review of patient safety practices that several colleagues and I conducted for the Agency for Healthcare Research and Quality, promoting the appropriate use VTE prophylaxis was the most highly rated practice on the strength of evidence regarding impact and effectiveness.[4]

PREVENTING PRESSURE ULCERS

Pressure ulcers, damage to skin or underlying structures caused by unrelieved pressure, cause pain, delay functional recovery, and predispose patients to local and systemic infections. It is estimated that about one in seven hospitalized patients has a pressure ulcer, that 2.5 million patients are treated for pressure ulcers each year in the United States alone, and that more than 50,000 patients die each year from their complications.[5,6]

Similar to patient falls (see "Preventing Falls," below), the first step in preventing pressure ulcers is identifying at-risk patients with a validated risk assessment tool. A variety of such tools are available—most assess nutritional status, mobility, incontinence, and sensory deficiencies. In the United States, the most commonly used tool is the Braden Scale.[7] Effective risk assessment involves an admission (to the hospital or skilled nursing facility) and subsequent (daily in hospitalized patients) assessments. These risk assessments are followed by a variety of preventive activities focused on at-risk patients. The Institute for Healthcare Improvement's (IHI) bundle recommends the following strategies: daily inspection of skin from head to toe (with a special focus on high-risk locations such as sacrum, buttocks, and heels), keeping the patient dry and treating overly dry skin with moisturizers, optimizing nutrition and hydration, and minimizing pressure through frequent turning and repositioning and the use of pressure relieving surfaces such as special beds. Several institutions have reported tremendous success in decreasing pressure ulcer rates through the systematic implementation of these risk assessment and mitigation strategies.[8,9]

PREVENTING FALLS

Patient falls are common—each year, more than one-third of community dwelling elders fall—and frequently morbid. As older patients are hospitalized or institutionalized, placed on multiple medications, and often immobilized, the risk for falls grows, with some studies suggesting that more than 50% of nursing home residents fall each year.[10] Injury rates are also higher in institutionalized patients, with approximately 20% of falls resulting in serious injury.[11] Interestingly, when asked about what they fear during a hospitalization, adult patients rate "falling and getting hurt" as a greater concern than "being misdiagnosed," "having the wrong test or procedure done," or "being mistaken for another patient," and only a bit below "errors with your medications" and "mistakes by nurses."[12]

All institutionalized patients should be assessed for fall risk with a validated instrument, such as the STRATIFY (St. Thomas risk assessment tool in falling elderly inpatients) tool[13] (Figure 11–1). In a validation study, patients with two or more fall risk factors on the STRATIFY tool had approximately a 50% chance of falling in the next week. In addition to the

---

STRATIFY risk assessment tool

---

1 Did the patient present to hospital with a fall or has he or she fallen in the ward since admission?

(Yes = 1, No = 0)

Do you think the patient is (questions 2–5)

2 Agitated?

(Yes = 1, No = 0)

3 Visually impaired to the extent that everyday function is affected?

(Yes = 1, No = 0)

4 In need of especially frequent toileting?

(Yes = 1, No = 0)

5 Transfer and mobility score of 3 or 4?

(Yes = 1, No = 0)

Total score = ▭

FIGURE 11–1. The STRATIFY risk assessment tool for falls. Transfer and mobility score is combination of Transfer score (0 = unable, 1 = major help needed, 2 = minor help, 3 = independent) and Mobility score (0 = immobile, 1= independent with aid of wheelchair, 2 = walks with help of one person, 3 = independent). Patients with two or more fall risk factors have a 50% chance of falling in the next week. (Reproduced with permission from Oliver D, Britton M, Seed P, et al. Development and evaluation of evidence based risk assessment tool (STRATIFY) to predict which elderly inpatients will fall: case-control and cohort studies. *BMJ* 1997;315:1049-1053.)

patient-centered risk factors captured in this tool, environmental (such as poor lighting and loose carpets) and extrinsic (such as polypharmacy) risk factors need to be considered[10] (Table 11–1). A recent systematic review found that the best predictors of future falls were a history of falls in the past year and the presence of active gait or balance problems.[14]

Particularly in patients found to be at risk for falls, active fall prevention efforts should be undertaken. Although the use of restraints (such as vests, bed rails, and wrist restraints) might appear to be a fall prevention strategy, emerging evidence suggests just the opposite.[15] For this reason (as well as for ethical reasons), restraints should be used as a fall prevention strategy only as a last resort. Other important strategies include early mobilization and efforts to preserve patient strength. Using hip protectors to

TABLE 11-1
Risk factors for patient falls in the hospital

- Fall as presenting complaint or history of falls
- Mobility impairment or unstable gait
- Muscle weakness
- Use of assistive devices
- Postural hypotension
- Visual deficits
- Cognitive impairment
- Agitation
- Urinary frequency
- Medications (e.g., psychotropics, class Ia antiarrhythmics, digoxin, and diuretics)
- Environmental factors (e.g., poor lighting, loose carpets)
- Arthritis
- Depression
- Age >80 years

Reproduced with permission from Bogardus ST. Another Fall. AHRQ WebM&M (serial online), April 2003. Available at: http://www. webmm.ahrq.gov/case.aspx?caseID=6.

prevent hip fractures in high-risk patients who do fall has shown benefit in some studies but not others.[16,17] A number of other commonsensical practices have also not been convincingly demonstrated to help, including the use of bed alarms to signal patient egress and the use of specially padded floors (which appear to decrease harm from falls but may increase fall risk from tripping). Although unstudied and challenging to implement, moving the mattress to the floor is an effective strategy for preventing harm from falls, particularly for confused patients who are apt to leave their bed.[10]

KEY POINTS

- As with healthcare-associated infections, several other complications of healthcare have been included under the patient safety umbrella. These include VTE, pressure ulcers, and patient falls.
- VTE guidelines are complex and rapidly changing. Improving adherence to appropriate prophylactic strategies depends on building

systems (including checklists and computerized decision support) to prompt their use.

- Many cases of pressure ulcers can be prevented by systematic risk assessment using validated tools, followed (particularly in at-risk patients) by extra attention to skin hygiene, nutrition and hydration, and avoiding undue pressure.

- Similarly, the approach to preventing falls begins with risk assessment, followed by strategies such as early mobilization, strength training, and lowering the mattress for at-risk patients.

REFERENCES

1. Shojania KG, Burton ED, McDonald KM, et al. Changes in rates of autopsy-detected diagnostic errors over time: a systematic review. *JAMA* 2003;289:2849–2856.

2. The Seventh ACCP Conference on Antithrombotic and Thrombolytic Therapy: Evidence-based Clinical Practice Guidelines. *Chest* 2004; 126(Suppl): 1S–92S.

3. Kucher N, Koo S, Quiroz R, et al. Electronic alerts to prevent venous thromboembolism among hospitalized patients. *N Engl J Med* 2005; 352:969–977.

4. Shojania KG, Duncan BW, McDonald KM, et al. Practices rated by strength of evidence. In: Shojania KG, Duncan BW, McDonald KM, et al., eds. *Making Health Care Safer: A Critical Analysis of Patient Safety Practices.* Evidence Report/Technology Assessment No. 43, AHRQ Publication No. 01-E058, 2001.

5. Lyder CH. Pressure ulcer prevention and management. *JAMA* 2003; 289:223–226.

6. Reddy M, Gill SS, Rochon PA. Preventing pressure ulcers: a systematic review. *JAMA* 2006;296:974–984.

7. Ayello EA, Braden B. How and why to do pressure ulcer risk assessment. *Adv Skin Wound Care* 2002;15:125–131; quiz 132–133.

8. Courtney BA, Ruppman JB, Cooper HM. Save our skin: initiative cuts pressure ulcer incidence in half. *Nurs Manage* 2006; 37:36, 38, 40 passim.

9. Gibbons W, Shanks HT, Kleinhelter P, et al. Eliminating facility-acquired pressure ulcers at Ascension Health. *Jt Comm J Qual Patient Saf* 2006; 32:488–496.

10. Bogardus ST. Another fall. AHRQ WebM&M (serial online), April 2003. Available at: http://www.webmm.ahrq.gov/case.aspx?caseID=6.

11. Rubenstein LZ, Josephson KR. Falls and their prevention in elderly people: what does the evidence show? *Med Clin North Am* 2006;90:807–824.

12. Burroughs TE, Waterman BM, Gallagher TH, et al. Patients' concerns about medical errors during hospitalization. *Jt Comm J Qual Improv* 2007;33:5–14.
13. Oliver D, Britton M, Seed P, et al. Development and evaluation of evidence based risk assessment tool (STRATIFY) to predict which elderly inpatients will fall: case-control and cohort studies. *BMJ* 1997;315:1049–1053.
14. Ganz DA, Bao Y, Shekelle PG, et al. Will my patient fall? *JAMA* 2007; 297:77–86.
15. Ejaz FK, Jones JA, Rose MS. Falls among nursing home residents: an examination of incident reports before and after restraint reduction programs. *J Am Geriatr Soc* 1994;42:960–964.
16. Agostini JV, Baker DI, Bogardus ST. Prevention of falls in hospitalized and institutionalized older people. In: Shojania KG, Duncan BW, McDonald KM, et al., eds. *Making Health Care Safer: A Critical Analysis of Patient Safety Practices.* Evidence Report/ Technology Assessment No. 43, AHRQ Publication No. 01-E058, 2001.
17. Kiel DP, Magaziner J, Zimmerman S, et al. Efficacy of a hip protector to prevent hip fracture in nursing home residents: the HIP PRO randomized controlled trial. *JAMA* 2007;298;413–422.

ADDITIONAL READINGS

Lyons SS. *Fall Prevention for Older Adults.* Iowa City, IA: University of Iowa Gerontological Nursing Interventions Research Center, Research Dissemination Core, 2004.

McGee DC, Gould MK. Preventing complications of central venous catheterization. *N Engl J Med* 2003;348:1123–1133.

National Center for Patient Safety Falls Toolkit 2004. Ann Arbor, MI: National Center for Patient Safety, 2004. Available at: http://www.patientsafety.gov/SafetyTopics/fallstoolkit/index.html.

Shojania KG, Duncan BW, McDonald KM, et al., eds. *Making Health Care Safer: A Critical Analysis of Patient Safety Practices.* Evidence Report/Technology Assessment No. 43, AHRQ Publication No. 01-E058, 2001.

CHAPTER TWELVE

Patient Safety in the Ambulatory Setting

GENERAL CONCEPTS AND EPIDEMIOLOGY

The point has been well made that while most of the patient safety literature comes from the hospital setting, most healthcare is delivered in office settings. Consider this: for every 1 hospitalized patient, 28 people visit a physician's office.[1] Nevertheless, the early emphasis on patient safety in the hospital was natural: the stakes are higher, errors are more visible, and the resources to research safety problems and implement solutions are all greater there. The scope of potential errors is also broader in the hospital—although both settings are beset by medication and laboratory errors, and most errors center around transitions of care and communication problems, the ambulatory setting will see fewer surgical errors (although the rapid increase in outpatient surgery makes these a growing problem) and health-care-associated infections, pressure ulcers, and blood clots are lesser concerns. Moreover, the research focus on hospital safety also reflects the disproportionate emphasis by academic health centers on hospital care.

But interest in ambulatory safety is growing rapidly, accompanied by a number of new research and practice initiatives. Recent studies have shown that nearly 10% of adverse events occur in physician offices[2]; adverse drug events and diagnostic errors are particularly common.[3,4] Early experience from new outpatient-based patient safety networks indicates that ambulatory practices should focus on two main areas: prescription medications and the processing of lab, x-ray, and diagnostic tests.[5,6]

This chapter will reflect on some of the differences between the hospital and the clinic that may impact efforts to improve safety in the latter setting.[7]

HOSPITAL VERSUS AMBULATORY ENVIRONMENTS

In the ambulatory world, the pace is slower and the rhythm more predictable (generally driven by a patient visit schedule) than in the hospital. The average error in the office is less consequential, because patients are less fragile and their medications and procedures are less potent (although the cumulative impact of errors may be surprisingly large because the volume is so high). In the hospital, much of the "action" centers around the patient's room—when the patient travels, the distances are relatively short (to the operating room, to radiology) and the patient remains within the same system. In the ambulatory environment, on the other hand, the patient may travel many miles to obtain a test or see a specialist, often entering and exiting practices that use different information systems and have vastly different clinical and operational styles and policies.

The structural and organizational differences may be even more important than the clinical ones. In all but the tiniest hospital, the scale is such that it is possible, indeed crucial, to employ individuals who specialize in the various tasks related to patient safety (Chapter 22). For example, even a modest size hospital is likely to have a quality officer, a compliance officer, a risk manager, and several information technology experts. A larger hospital will have armies of people in these departments, and may even employ a human factors specialist and a patient safety officer. In the average small office practice, a physician (or nurse or practice administrator) will wear all of these hats. Moreover, because none of these specialized staff members generate patient care revenue, the ability of a small practice to support them is far more limited than in the hospital (they do not produce revenue in the hospital either, but they can be cross-subsidized by lucrative activities that do). Office practice is less highly regulated, and, because most of the care takes place behind closed doors (with just doctor and patient in the room), it is easier for errors to avoid the light of day. Even the cultural issues (Chapters 9 and 15) have a very different flavor. For example, consider programs that aim to improve physician-nurse relationships and diminish the steep authority gradients that are often present. In American hospitals (where the physician is likely to be self-employed while the nurse works for the hospital), the shape of such programs is likely to be very different than in the office (where the doctor will frequently be the nurse's employer).

Many of these differences would appear to favor the hospital as an environment to establish a flourishing patient safety enterprise. However, the ambulatory setting also has some unique advantages. First, simplification, standardization, and the implementation of information technology may yield more palpable efficiency advantages. When a single clerk or nurse is working with three physicians in an office practice, the impact of getting each of these physicians to agree on standard procedures for following up lab results is often profound. And the office space freed up by converting to a paperless medical record system can yield major economic advantages for a practice. Second, efforts to engage patients in helping to ensure their own safety are more likely to be productive (Chapter 21), because ambulatory patients are less apt to be mentally slowed by their disease or medications or distracted by anxiety. In addition, ambulatory patients are better able to intervene (because there are fewer tests and procedures and the pace is slower) when they see something out of place. The previously mentioned organizational structure of most American practices can become another advantage. In many hospitals, the doctors are not particularly invested in the safety enterprise (because they use the hospital to provide care but don't own the organization), whereas most office practices in the United States are owned by the physicians themselves. The old saying, "nobody ever washed a rented car" helps explain the challenge faced by those who try to engage office-based physicians in hospital safety efforts (Chapter 22).

Overall, the implications of the ambulatory versus hospital differences will be important to appreciate as we increasingly turn our attention to outpatient safety. Most ambulatory practices will be able to identify a relatively small number of common but risky practices to focus their safety efforts on, such as medication prescribing, follow-up of laboratory and x-ray test results, and communication with referring physicians and hospital providers. The implementation of information technology systems is likely to be highly disruptive to the practice but may quickly yield tangible benefits.[8] The relative absence of outside scrutiny by regulators, legislators, and the media will necessitate other motivations, including providers' professionalism and commitment to their patients. Efforts to improve culture will often need to take into account the employer-employee relationship.

Overall, improving safety in the ambulatory setting will not necessarily be harder or easier than in the hospital, just different. As with much of the patient safety field, which involves extrapolating experiences from other settings (i.e., Will Crew-Resource Management, which worked so well in commercial aviation, work in the labor and delivery suite? Will bar coding, which works so well in the supermarket, actually decrease

---

TABLE 12–1

Practices that may lead to improved ambulatory medication safety

Write understandable, legible prescriptions, and include the indication on the prescription. Use English instead of Latin abbreviations (i.e., writing "four times daily" or "once daily" instead of "qid" and "qd," respectively), and write the indication on the prescription (e.g., "for high blood pressure").

Use sample medications with care, if at all. Pharmacists serve as an important safety check when prescribing medications, often catching interactions and allergies that physicians miss.

Maintain accurate and usable medication lists and reconcile medications regularly. Use the "brown bag check-up" (i.e., ask patients to bring all the medicines in their medicine cabinet to a visit). Physicians and their staff need to confirm the medications at every visit. When discrepancies are found, it is the physician's task to resolve these.

Empower patients to serve as safety double-checkers. Most patients can assume significant responsibility for discovering—and preventing—many medical errors from becoming harmful events.

Consider using an electronic prescribing system. An electronic prescribing system, especially when interfaced with an electronic health record, has the potential to decrease errors from illegibility and interactions. Direct electronic transmission to pharmacies may decrease errors even further.

Reproduced with permission from Elder NC. Patient safety in the physician office setting. AHRQ WebM&M (serial online), May 2006. Available at: http://webmm.ahrq.gov/perspective.aspx? perspectiveID=24.

medication errors?), it will be important to remain sensitive to the differences in structure and culture as we try to translate what we know about hospital safety to the office setting. Elder has suggested a number of commonsense practices that may lead to improvements in ambulatory medication safety (Table 12–1) and management of test results (Table 12–2).

KEY POINTS

- Up until recently, the patient safety field's focus has been on hospital safety. Attention is now shifting to the ambulatory setting.
- Efforts to improve ambulatory safety should initially focus on decreasing medication errors and improving the management of test results.

TABLE 12-2

Practices that may lead to improved ambulatory management of test results

Implement a formal test-tracking system. A tracking system assures that all tests ordered are returned, ideally to the physician but at least to the practice. Although a formal tracking system can be incorporated within an electronic health record, this is not a requirement for having a working system. A system needs to be simple, have some built-in redundancies (to account for human error in entering data), and be accessible and accountable to multiple people (not just "Mary in the laboratory"). An electronic results manager can track results and provide reminders.

Make a policy of notifying every patient of every result. "No news is good news" should be a policy relegated to history. Practices should decide on a standard ized system for notifying patients of both normal and abnormal results.

Empower patients to serve as safety double-checks. Patients should be educated as to what tests are being ordered, their purpose, and when (and how) results will be relayed. If patients do not receive their results within a specified time, they should be instructed to contact the office for the results.

Only file signed reports, letters, dictations, and results. Whereas many offices have a policy that nothing enters a chart (electronic or paper) without being signed first, too often, unsigned or inappropriately signed reports get filed. The response to the report (normal, abnormal) also needs to be noted by the physician.

Reproduced with permission from Elder NC. Patient safety in the physician office setting. AHRQ WebM&M (serial online), May 2006. Available at: http://webmm.ahrq.gov/perspective.aspx?perspectiveID=24.

- In approaching ambulatory safety, it will be important to appreciate major clinical, structural, and organizational differences between the hospital and the office. These include the inability to support specialized experts in many safety-related areas, and the employer-employee relationship between physicians and many nurses and other staff found in most office practices in the United States.

REFERENCES

1. Green LA, Fryer GE, Yawn BP, et al. The ecology of medical care revisited. *N Engl J Med* 2001;344:2021–2025.
2. Weingart SN, Wilson RM, Gibberd RW, et al. Epidemiology of medical error. *BMJ* 2000;320:774–777.

3. Gandhi TK, Weingart SN, Borus J, et al. Adverse drug events in ambulatory care. *N Engl J Med* 2003;348:1556–1564.
4. Gandhi TK, Kachalia A, Thomas EJ, et al. Missed and delayed diagnoses in the ambulatory setting: a study of closed malpractice claims. *Ann Intern Med* 2006;145:488–496.
5. Elder NC. Patient safety in the physician office setting. AHRQ WebM&M (serial online), May 2006. Available at: http://webmm.ahrq.gov/perspective. aspx?perspectiveID=24.
6. West D, Westfall JM, Araya-Guerra R, et al. Using reported primary care errors to develop and implement patient safety interventions: a report from the ASIPS Collaborative. In: *Advances in Patient Safety: From Research to Implementation*. Rockville, MD: Agency for Healthcare Research and Quality, 2005, AHRQ Publication No. 050021.
7. Wachter RM. Is ambulatory patient safety just like hospital safety, only without the "stat?" *Ann Intern Med* 2006;145:547–549.
8. Baron RJ, Fabens EL, Schiffman M, et al. Electronic health records: just around the corner? Or over the cliff? *Ann Intern Med* 2005;143:222–226.

ADDITIONAL READINGS

Bhasale AL, Miller GC, Reid SE, et al. Analysing potential harm in Australian general practice: an incident-monitoring study. *Med J Aust* 1998;169:73–76.

Gandhi TK, Weingart SN, Seger AC, et al. Outpatient prescribing errors and the impact of computerized prescribing. *J Gen Intern Med* 2005;20:837–841.

Gurwitz JH, Field TS, Harrold LR, et al. Incidence and preventability of adverse drug events among older persons in the ambulatory setting. *JAMA* 2003;289:1107–1116.

Nassaralla CL, Naessens JM, Chaudhry R, et al. Implementation of a medication reconciliation process in an ambulatory internal medicine clinic. *Qual Saf Health Care* 2007;16:90–94.

Poon EG, Gandhi TK, Sequist TD, et al. "I wish I had seen this test result earlier!" Dissatisfaction with test result management systems in primary care. *Arch Intern Med* 2004;164: 2223–2228.

Schauberger CW, Larson P. Implementing patient safety practices in small ambulatory care settings. *Jt Comm J Qual Patient Saf* 2006; 32:419–425.

Solutions

CHAPTER THIRTEEN

Information Technology

HEALTHCARE'S INFORMATION PROBLEM

The provision of healthcare is remarkably information intensive. A large integrated healthcare system will process many more computerized transactions each day (10 million or so) than the NASDAQ stock exchange (2 million).

But volume only begins the challenge. Consider the task of tracking a single patient's current diseases, past medical history, medications, allergies, test results, risk factors, and personal preferences (such as for cardiopulmonary resuscitation). Tricky? Sure, but now do it over months or years, and then add in the fact that the patient is seen by many different providers, scattered across a region. Want more? To make payment decisions, the insurer needs access to some of this information, as does the source of the insurance, which in the United States is often the patient's employer. But, because of privacy concerns, both should only receive essential information; to tell them of the patient's HIV status, or her psychiatric or sexual history, would be highly inappropriate, damaging, and possibly illegal.

Now let's make it really hard. Assume that the patient is in a car accident and taken to an emergency department (ED) in a nearby state, where she is stabilized and admitted to the hospital. Ideally, the doctors and nurses would see the relevant clinical details of her past history, preferably in a format that highlighted the information they needed without overwhelming them with extraneous data. Orders must be processed instantaneously (none of "the system is down for planned maintenance" or "orders are processed on the next business day" so familiar from commercial transactions). During her hospital stay, not only would there be seamless linkages among all of the new observations (the neurosurgeon can easily view the ED doctor's notes; the resident can quickly find the patient's vital signs and laboratory studies), but the various components would weave together seamlessly. For example:

- The system would prompt the doctor with information regarding the appropriate therapy or test for a given condition (along with links to the evidence supporting any recommendations).

- The system would warn the nurse that the patient is allergic to a medicine before she administers it.

- The system would tell the doctor or pharmacist which medications are on the formulary and steer them to the preferred ones.

Meanwhile, the vast treasure trove of data being created through this patient's encounter—and millions of others like it—would be chronicled and analyzed ("mined"), searching for new patterns of disease, evidence of preferred strategies, and more. All of this would be iterative—as new information emerged from this and other research about risk factors for diseases or best practices, it would seamlessly flow into the system, guiding the next patient's care to be even better.

Contrast this vision of information nirvana to the prevailing state of most doctors' offices and hospitals. Information is stored on paper charts, and thus unavailable to anyone who lacks physical possession of the relevant piece of paper (in some cases, the notes are sufficiently illegible that even physical custody of the paper does not insure information access). Notes are entered as free text, not in a format that facilitates analysis or productive interaction with other pieces of system data. When the patient moves across silos—from outpatient to inpatient, from state to state, from hospital to hospice—the necessary information is unlikely to move with her. Communication of facts (e.g., medication lists, allergies, past medical history), which should be streamed through the system, instead lives at the mercy of person-to-person interactions or a haphazard pinball game of photocopies bouncing from place to place.

Even at the level of the individual practitioner, the impact of this chaos is profoundly demoralizing and wasteful. Just watch a nurse take a patient's vital signs on a typical hospital ward. The nurse looks at the numbers on the screen of a digital automated blood pressure cuff: **165/92**. She records them on an index card (or, sometimes, on her skin or the cuff of her scrub suit), hopefully next to the correct patient's name. Later, she returns to the nurses' station and transcribes these numbers (again, hopefully belonging to the correct patient) onto the appropriate place in the chart (hopefully the right chart). Then, in a teaching hospital, an intern transcribes these vital signs onto another index card during morning rounds. He presents this data to his resident and later to his attending, who each do the same thing. Eventually, each of these practitioners writes, or dictates, notes for the medical record. Any wonder that this information (which, you'll recall, began life in digital form!) is frequently wrong? Or that busy healthcare professionals find that huge amounts of their valuable time is squandered? Or that the patient has the sense (particularly after she has been asked the same question by 10 different people) that the right hand has no idea what the left hand is doing?

Why has healthcare, the most information-intensive of industries, failed to enter the modern age of computers? Part of the reason is that, up until recently, the business or clinical case for healthcare information technology (HIT) was far from ironclad. Such justification was needed because HIT is extraordinarily expensive (estimated at about 50,000 dollars per doctor in an ambulatory office, and up to 100 million dollars to completely wire a large teaching hospital), unreimbursed, and extremely challenging to implement. Moreover, until the past few years, most healthcare computer systems were relatively clunky and user unfriendly, in part because the market for them was too weak to fund the research and development—and to propel the user feedback and refinement cycles—needed for complex systems to mature.

All of this has begun to change, as a growing body of literature now demonstrates the benefits of well-designed and implemented electronic systems.[1-4] We appear, finally, to be entering the age of healthcare computerization, catalyzed in large part by the perceived benefits to patient safety and by widespread promotion of HIT by a broad range of stakeholders (Chapter 20). This chapter will describe the main types of HIT systems, some of their safety advantages (Table 13–1), and some of the problems—including new kinds of errors—they can create.[5-7]

TABLE 13–1

Mechanisms by which information technology can improve patient safety

- Improving communication
- Making knowledge more readily accessible
- Prompting for key pieces of information
- Assisting with calculations
- Monitoring and checking in real time
- Providing decision support

Reproduced with permission from Bates DW, Gawande AA. Improving safety with information technology. *N Engl J Med* 2003;348:2526-2534.

ELECTRONIC MEDICAL RECORDS

Because most medical errors represent failures in communication and data transmission (Figure 9–4), computerization of the medical record would seem like a safety lynchpin. But to realize this benefit, attention needs to be paid to a variety of system and user factors. The system factors include the ease of use, the speed with which data can be entered and retrieved, the quality of the user interface, and the presence of value-added features such as order entry, decision support, sign-out and scheduling systems, links to all the necessary data (e.g., x-rays and electrocardiograms), and automatic reports. The user factors primarily relate to the training and readiness of the provider and nonprovider workforce (Chapters 7 and 16).

User efficiency is particularly important. Despite the promise by many information technology proponents that computerization would save time for providers, emerging evidence indicates that the opposite is often true, particularly for physicians.[8] Some of this cost in time is repaid by more efficient information retrieval, but increasing attention will need to be paid to facilitating provider workflow (remember that digital blood pressure reading—in the "wired" hospital, it will magically leap from blood pressure machine into the electronic medical record, where it can be seamlessly imported into each provider's note). Effective systems will, of course, provide huge efficiency benefits to administrators, researchers, and insurers by capturing data in more standardized formats and allowing electronic transmission.

Unfortunately, this facilitated movement of bits and bytes has a dark side, in the form of the "copy and paste" phenomenon. One tongue-in-cheek essayist captured the problem beautifully:

> The copy-and-paste command allows one day's note to be copied and used as a template for the next day's note. Ideally, old information and diagnostic impressions are deleted and new ones added. In reality, however, there is no deletion, only addition. Daily progress notes become progressively longer and contain senescent information. The admitting diagnostic impression, long since discarded, is dutifully noted day after day. Last month's echocardiogram report takes up permanent residence in the daily results section. Complicated patients are on "post-op day 2" for weeks. One wonders how utilization review interprets such statements.[9]

A study of 167,000 computerized records in the United States Department of Veterans Affairs (VA) healthcare system found that physical examinations were completely copied (from one author to another) in 3% of the charts.[10] Like many elements of patient safety, introducing an electronic medical record without the requisite education and professionalism is likely to lead to new types of patient harm.

COMPUTERIZED PROVIDER ORDER ENTRY

Because the prescribing process is one of the Achilles' heels of medication safety (Figure 4–3), efforts to computerize this process have long been a focus of safety efforts. Bates and colleagues demonstrated that a computerized provider order entry (CPOE) system with decision support reduced serious medication errors by 55%, mediated by improved communication, better availability of information, constraints to prevent the use of inappropriate drugs, doses, and frequencies, and assistance with monitoring.[2,11] A later study of more sophisticated decision support found an 83% reduction in medication errors.[12] The advantages of CPOE over paper-based system are many (Table 13–2); in addition to those listed in the table, the installation of CPOE systems inevitably leads organizations to standardize chaotic processes (the equivalent of cleaning out your closet before moving), which has its own safety advantages.[2]

Much of the value of CPOE systems comes from identifying out-of-range results or potentially unsafe interactions, and rapidly alerting providers so that they can decide whether their plan is correct. For example, a CPOE system can alert a provider to a potentially fatal medication-allergy interaction (Figure 13–1) or a potentially dangerous laboratory result (Table 13–3). These systems can also be used at the healthcare system level to identify and track errors ("trigger tools") (Chapter 14).

In addition to helping clinicians avoid mistakes, CPOE systems can also suggest actions that should always accompany certain orders. These *"corollary orders"* should be second nature, but our memories are fallible and we will sometimes forget to check a creatinine and potassium after starting an angiotensin-converting enzyme (ACE) inhibitor, a digoxin level after beginning digoxin, or a glucose level after starting insulin. In one study, clinicians were twice as likely to accept a computerized prompt of a corollary order than they were to order the level without the prompting.[13]

TABLE 13-2

Advantages of CPOE systems over paper-based systems

- Free of handwriting identification problems
- Faster to reach the pharmacy
- Less subject to error associated with similar drug names
- More easily integrated into medical records and decision support systems
- Less subject to errors caused by use of apothecary measures
- Easily linked to drug-drug interaction warnings
- More likely to identify the prescribing physician
- Able to link to ADE reporting systems
- Able to avoid specification errors, such as trailing zeros
- Available and appropriate for training and education
- Available for immediate data analysis, including postmarketing reporting
- Claimed to generate significant economic savings
- With online prompts, CPOE systems can:

    Link to algorithms to emphasize cost-effective medications

    Reduce underprescribing and overprescribing

    Reduce incorrect drug choices

Abbreviation: ADE, adverse drug event.

Reproduced with permission from Koppel R, Metlay JP, Cohen A, et al. Role of computerized physician order entry systems in facilitating medication errors. *JAMA* 2005;293:1197-1203.

Despite the great appeal of CPOE, one study at an academic medical center found 22 new error types caused or exacerbated by a commercial CPOE system, including long gaps in medication delivery because of a fragmented CPOE display, failure to discontinue medications or renew antibiotics, and delayed ordering caused by CPOE system downtime.[5] Even more concerning, one study found a threefold *increase* in the mortality rate of critically ill pediatric patients after a new CPOE system was installed.[6] There, caregivers noted inefficient order entry, too much time spent at the computer screen and away from the bedside, and several other problems in workflow.

These cautionary notes are all relatively recent—earlier studies of computerization were uniformly positive.[11-13] But these initial studies came from a handful of early adopter institutions that built homegrown systems

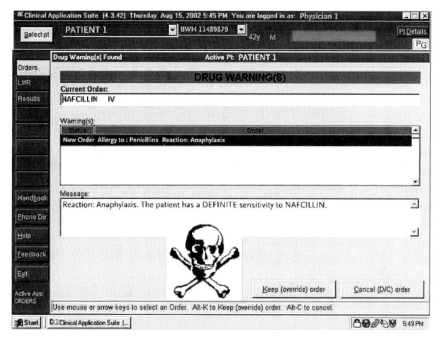

FIGURE 13–1. Example of a CPOE system's warning of a potentially fatal medication-allergy interaction. (Reproduced with permission from Bates DW, Gawande AA. Improving safety with information technology. *N Engl J Med* 2003; 348: 2526-2534.)

over decades, supported by skilled and highly committed informaticians, researchers, and leaders. As we wrote in *Internal Bleeding,*

> But the average hospital will not share these conditions, any more than your local Gilbert and Sullivan troupe resembles the Metropolitan Opera . . . More than one CIO has tried to airlift a commercial system into her hospital, then stood scratching her head at how slick the system seemed to be during the vendor's demo, and how poorly it performed in real life.[14]

We can expect that, as the market for CPOE grows and commercial products go through many crucial user-generated improvement cycles, the systems will become better, errors associated with them will become less common, and the full safety benefits of CPOE will begin to be realized.

TABLE 13-3
Sample critical laboratory values*

Lab Test	Critical Values		Common Qualifications or Variations
	Low	High	
Serum glucose	<40 or 45 mg/dL	>500 mg/dL	High value could have lower threshold in newborns (e.g., >200 mg/dL)
Serum sodium	<120 meq/L	>160 meq/L	High value could have lower threshold (e.g., >152 meq/L)
Serum potassium	<2.5 meq/L	>6.0 meq/L	Either value could have slightly different threshold
Serum bicarbonate	≤10 meq/L	≥40 meq/L	Either value could have slightly different threshold
Serum calcium (total)	<7.0 mg/dL	>13.0 mg/dL	Either value could have slightly different threshold
White blood cell count	$<2 \times 10^{-9}$/L	$>50 \times 10^{-9}$/L	Low value could be specified in terms of absolute neutrophil count (e.g., ANC $<0.5 \times 10^{-9}$/L). High value could have threshold as high as 100×10^{-9}/L. Thresholds commonly vary across settings (inpatient vs. outpatient) and patient populations (oncology patients, pediatrics)
Hematocrit	<20%	>60%	Inpatient settings often omit critical threshold for high values
Platelet count	$<20 \times 10^{-9}$/L	$>1000 \times 10^{-9}$/L	Threshold for low value commonly varies across settings (inpatient vs. outpatient) and patient populations (oncology patients, pediatrics)
Prothrombin time	Not applicable	International normalized ratio (INR) > 5	

Partial thromboplastin time	Not applicable	>100 s	High value may have higher threshold (e.g., >120 s) or may be specified relative to the normal range (e.g., >3 times upper limit of normal)
Blood culture	Not applicable	Positive result	
Cerebrospinal fluid culture or direct examination	Not applicable	Positive result	
Acid fast bacilli stain (any specimen)	Not applicable	Positive result	

*A typical policy for the appropriate response to a critical value is that someone from the laboratory must notify by telephone a physician, nurse, physician assistant, or medical assistant at the ordering location. In accordance with Joint Commission requirements, laboratory staff must ask the recipient of the results to read back the results to ensure that the results were properly received. (Reproduced with permission from Astion M. The result stopped here. AHRQ WebM&M (serial online), June 2004. Available at: http://webmm.ahrq.gov/case.aspx?caseID=65).

OTHER IT-RELATED SAFETY SOLUTIONS

Bar Coding and Radiofrequency Identification Systems

Even when rigorous safety checks are embedded into the prescribing process, errors at the time of drug administration can still lead to great harm (Chapter 4). To prevent these errors, many institutions are implementing bar coding or radiofrequency identification (RFID) solutions. In bar code medication administration (BCMA), a nurse must swipe a bar code on the medication, the patient's wristband, and her own badge to confirm a three-way match before a medication can be administered.[15] In RFID systems, the medication package has an implanted chip that transmits a signal, allowing for passive identification (like driving through an automated toll booth) rather than requiring a scan. Despite its intuitive appear, RFID remains more expensive, and—because patients are taking multiple medications and nurses often have the medications for multiple patients on their carts—somewhat trickier to implement.

Like all HIT systems, BCMA has its challenges. Nurses worry that it will take too much time—and some observers have already documented workarounds (such as when a nurse takes a handful of patient wristbands and scans them outside the patient's room to save time) that bypass the systems' safety features. Another concern is whether BCMA systems can be sufficiently flexible when patients are acutely ill.[15,16] Finally, BCMA must be rooted in an environment of robust safety processes. We documented one case in which two patients (one a poorly controlled diabetic) were mistakenly given each other's bar coded wristbands, nearly leading to a fatal insulin overdose in the nondiabetic whose glucose checks erroneously indicated that he had a stratospheric blood sugar.[7] Like all IT systems, BCMA can become a very efficient error propagator if the inputted data are incorrect. These concerns notwithstanding, effective use of BCMA technology can substantially reduce medication dispensing errors,[17] and its popularity is likely to grow in the coming years.

Smart Intravenous Pumps

Progress in medication safety through BCMA still leaves a large gap: the safety of medications infused intravenously. Approximately 90% of hospitalized patients receive at least one intravenous medication. Because many of these medications are far more dangerous than pills, and their doses are more variable (often calculated by the hour, or through complex weight- and size-based formulae), the opportunity for harm is real, particularly as errors at the administration phase leave no opportunity to be "caught." Because of this, there has been considerable interest in so-called "smart intravenous pumps."

Smart pumps are engineered to have built-in danger alerts, clinical calculators, and drug libraries that include information on the standard concentrations of frequently used drugs. They also can record every infusion, creating a database that can identify risky situations and medications for future interventions. Studies have shown that these pumps can prevent many infusion errors,[18–20] but that increasing attention has to be paid to seamlessly interfacing these systems with other computerized medication systems such as CPOE and BCMA.[21] When one considers the increasing number and complexity of intravenous infusions in hospitalized (Figure 13–2), and now even homebound, patients, perfecting this technology should be a high priority.

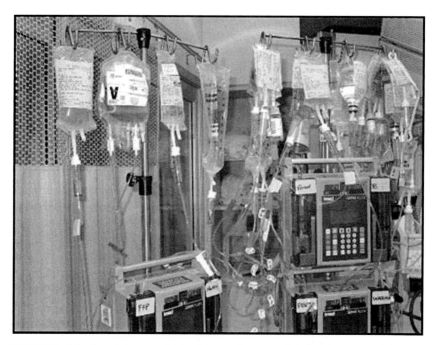

FIGURE 13–2.   A not-atypical picture of a sea of IV bags in a modern ICU. (Reproduced with permission from Michael Gropper, MD, PhD)

Other IT Solutions

When people think of information technology and patient safety, they generally think of electronic medical records, computerized order entry, and perhaps BCMA. However, it is worth pointing out that a wide range of other information-system-based solutions can help improve safety. For example, in many hospitals, staff members now wear voice-activated wireless microphones, or use modern text paging or cell phone systems, to facilitate instant communication between caregivers. The value of IT-based sign-out systems and computer-based simulation is discussed in Chapters 8 and 17, respectively. And we shouldn't forget the importance of more clinically oriented HIT, such as the Picture Archiving and Communication Systems (PACS) that allow digital radiographs to be reviewed from a few miles, or a few thousand miles, away from the hospital.[22] In addition to their convenience, PACS can decrease x-ray interpretation errors by facilitating double reads, computerized enhancements of images, and access to prior radiographs.[23] Moving even closer to the patient, the use of handheld ultrasound can lower the risks of central-line placement or thoracentesis.[24,25]

COMPUTERIZED DECISION SUPPORT

Although much of HIT's emphasis has been on replacing the paper chart and moving information around, the ultimate value may lie mainly in computerized decision support. Once clinical care is computerized, it becomes possible to provide information to clinicians at the point of care. For example, some systems provide simple alerts such as drug-drug, drug-allergy, or drug-lab interactions (Figure 13–1), or links to evidence-based guidelines (the clinician types in a diagnosis of "pneumonia" and a link to a recent pneumonia management guideline materializes).

But that is just the start. More prescriptive decision support systems can "hard wire" certain kinds of care. For example, order sets for common diagnoses can be loaded into a CPOE system, "making it easy to do the right thing" by simply clicking a few boxes.[4,26] Or an intensive care unit (ICU) system can alert the physician or nurse when a patient's vital signs go outside preset parameters (Figure 13–3). Note that these prescriptive systems usually permit clinicians to deviate from recommended protocols, but this takes more time (because the doctor needs to type out the

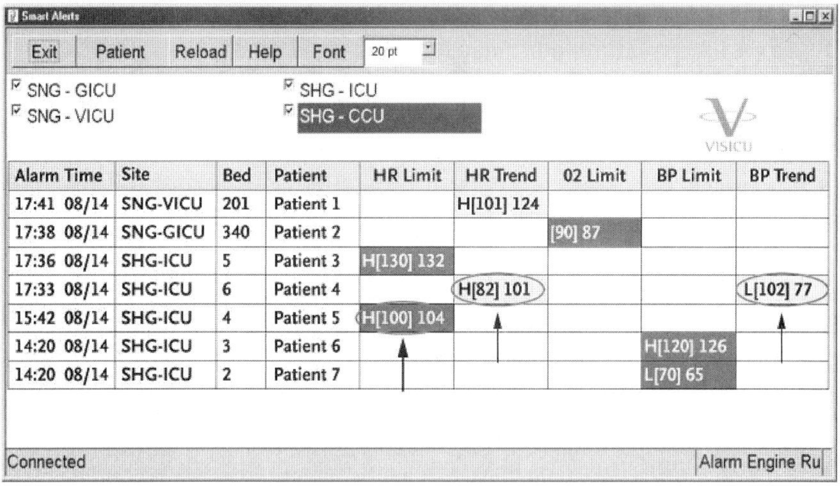

FIGURE 13–3. "Smart" monitoring system in an ICU. This screen highlights physiologic changes that are occurring (in this case, a rapid pulse and a trend toward increasing pulse and decreasing blood pressure [BP]); such monitoring can help clinicians to detect and respond to such changes before an adverse event occurs. The heart-rate (HR) limit alert is triggered when the heart rate crosses a high (H) or low (L) limit, which are determined according to the patient's active medical conditions. Patient 5 (thick arrow) has had surgery and is at risk for perioperative coronary events. The limit value is given in brackets, followed by the patient's current value. The heart-rate or blood-pressure trend alert is triggered if the heart rate or blood pressure changes substantially over a period of several hours. Patient 4 (thin arrows) has an increasing heart rate and a decreasing blood pressure; on evaluation, this patient was found to have hypovolemia. The baseline value is given in brackets, followed by the current value. (Reproduced with permission from Bates DW, Gawande AA. Improving safety with information technology. *N Engl J Med* 2003;348:2526–2534.)

orders instead of accepting an order set, and may even be asked to state or check the reason for deviation). Even more prescriptively, the computer could all-but-force a given practice, making the clinician jump through several hoops (such as "call a specialist for approval") before being allowed to deviate.

IT SOLUTIONS FOR IMPROVING DIAGNOSTIC ACCURACY

Finally, another type of decision support focuses on improving diagnostic accuracy (Chapter 6). Early clinical artificial intelligence programs— in which clinicians entered key elements from the history, physical examination, and laboratory studies and the computer fashioned a list of diagnosis—were disappointing, because the computer-generated diagnostic lists mixed plausible possibilities with nonsensical ones, and the data entry time (over and above clinical charting time) was prohibitive.[27] Recent advances have generated new interest in diagnostic decision support. For example, some programs now pull data directly from the electronic medical record, bypassing the need for redundant data entry. Others mine textbooks and journal articles to find diagnoses most frequently associated with citations of certain symptoms and signs.[28] Most modern programs not only suggest possible diagnoses but link to helpful resources and references. One can envision future computerized decision aides that draw their source information from the electronic medical record, produce possible diagnoses that are automatically updated with new information, and actually "learn" by integrating prior experiences from the system itself, making them ever-more-accurate over time.

THE CHALLENGES OF COMPUTERIZATION

Although one might see all of this as terribly exciting—and it is—the computerization of healthcare is also brimming with challenges. Systems that opt to be less prescriptive, perhaps focusing on providing physicians with additional information rather than forcing certain practices, will generally depend on "alerts" that pop up in the process of care. These can result in *alert fatigue*, as clinicians rapidly tire of the alerts and fail to notice even important ones. For example, one study of approximately 5000 computerized alerts showed that clinicians overrode "critical drug interaction" and "allergy-drug interaction" alerts in approximately three out of four cases.[29] And these alerts may anger clinicians—in one famous case, an expensive CPOE system failed in part because physicians rebelled against all the alerts.[30] As systems become more prescriptive, clinicians may bristle at the hardwired care protocols, especially if they appear to lack the necessary flexibility ("*cookbook medicine*"). Diagnostic decision support systems are likely to be judged on the seamlessness of the inputting process (the best will be those that draw their inputs directly from the electronic record) and the plausibility and helpfulness of the diagnostic possibilities emanating from the system. As of yet, few studies convincingly demonstrating that these systems improve patient outcomes or diagnostic accuracy.

On the other hand, given the frequency of non-evidence-based medicine and the high prevalence of diagnostic errors, it is difficult to argue that computerized decision support and other HIT solutions should not be aggressively researched and promoted. At this point, despite the emerging evidence of benefit and the promotion of HIT by payer coalitions and others (Chapter 20), adoption of CPOE and the electronic medical record has been remarkably slow. As of 2007, only about 15% of U.S. hospitals had fully adopted CPOE, an adoption curve far slower than that of other technologies such as the VCR, the Internet, and e-mail. The obstacles are many, including financial (particularly if the cost is borne by physicians and hospitals and many of the benefits accrue to insurers), the relative absence of standards (which inhibits interoperability of systems and opportunities for users to switch products over time), and the cultural barriers described above.[2,31]

As these barriers are overcome and pressure grows to meet publicly reported quality and safety standards (Chapter 3), the adoption of HIT is likely to skyrocket. As with so much else in patient safety, the key to the success of clinical IT systems will be careful design and implementation, because even information technology systems can create harm as well as benefit.

KEY POINTS

- The implementation of HIT has been remarkably slow until recently, but the pace is beginning to accelerate.

- Many healthcare activities require multiple providers (and others) to view (legible) patient-level information simultaneously, a powerful argument for electronic medical records.

- CPOE can ensure that physicians' orders are legible and respect preset parameters.

- Bar coding or other similar systems can help decrease the frequency of medication administration (and other patient identification-related) errors.

- Ultimately, much of the benefit of HIT will come through the thoughtful implementation of computerized decision support, which ranges from simply providing information to clinicians at the point of care to more prescriptive systems that "hardwire" certain elements of care.

REFERENCES

1. Jha AK, Poon EG, Bates DW, et al. Defining the priorities and challenges for the adoption of Information Technology in HealthCare: opinions from an expert panel. *AMIA Annu Symp Proc* 2003;2003:881.
2. Bates DW, Gawande AA. Improving safety with information technology. *N Engl J Med* 2003;348:2526–2534.
3. Rothschild JM, Keohane CA, Cook EF, et al. A controlled trial of smart infusion pumps to improve medication safety in critically ill patients. *Crit Care Med* 2005;33:533–540.
4. Kucher N, Koo S, Quiroz R, et al. Electronic alerts to prevent venous thromboembolism among hospitalized patients. *N Engl J Med* 2005;352: 969–977.
5. Koppel R, Metlay JP, Cohen A, et al. Role of computerized physician order entry systems in facilitating medication errors. *JAMA* 2005;293:1197–1203.
6. Han YY, Carcillo JA, Venkataraman ST, et al. Unexpected increased mortality after implementation of a commercially sold computerized physician order entry system. *Pediatrics* 2005;116:1506–1512.
7. McDonald CJ. Computerization can create safety hazards: a bar-coding near miss. *Ann Intern Med* 2006;144:510–516.
8. Poissant L, Pereira J, Tamblyn R, et al. The impact of electronic health records on time efficiency of physicians and nurses: a systematic review. *Am Med Inform Assoc* 2005;12:505–516.
9. Hirschtick RE. A piece of my mind. Copy-and-paste. *JAMA* 2006; 295:2335–2336.
10. Thielke S, Hammond K, Helbig S. Copying and pasting of examinations within the electronic medical record. *Int J Med Inform* 2006.
11. Bates DW, Leape LL, Cullen DJ, et al. Effect of computerized physician order entry and a team intervention on prevention of serious medication errors. *JAMA* 1998;280:1311–1316.
12. Bates DW, Teich JM, Lee J, et al. The impact of computerized physician order entry on medication error prevention. *J Am Med Inform Assoc* 1999; 6:313–321.
13. Overhage JM, Tierney WM, Zhou XH, et al. A randomized trial of "corollary orders" to prevent errors of omission. *J Am Med Inform Assoc* 1997;4:364–375.
14. Wachter RM, Shojania KG. *Internal Bleeding: The Truth Behind America's Terrifying Epidemic of Medical Mistakes*. New York, NY: Rugged Land, 2004.
15. Wright AA, Katz IT. Bar coding for patient safety. *N Engl J Med* 2005; 454:329–331.
16. Patterson ES, Cook RI, Render ML. Improving patient safety by identifying side effects from introducing bar coding in medication administration. *J Am Med Inform Assoc* 2002;9:540–553.

17. Poon EG, Cina JL, Churchill W, et al. Medication dispensing errors and potential adverse drug events before and after implementing bar code technology in the pharmacy. *Ann Intern Med* 2006;145:426–434.

18. Keohane CA, Hayes J, Saniuk C, et al. Intravenous medication safety and smart infusion systems: lessons learned and future opportunities. *J Infus Nurs* 2005;28:321–328.

19. Larsen GY, Parker HB, Cash J, et al. Standard drug concentrations and smart-pump technology reduce continuous-medication-infusion errors in pediatric patients. *Pediatrics* 2005;116:e21–e25.

20. Williams CK, Maddox RR, Heape E, et al. Application of the IV Medication Harm Index to assess the nature of harm averted by "smart" infusion safety systems. *J Patient Saf* 2006;2:132–139.

21. Husch M, Sullivan C, Rooney D, et al. Insights from the sharp end of intravenous medication errors: implications for infusion pump technology. *Qual Saf Health Care* 2005;14:80–86.

22. Wachter RM. International teleradiology. *N Engl J Med* 2006;354: 662–663.

23. Bryan S, Weatherburn G, Buxton M, et al. Evaluation of a hospital picture archiving and communication system. *J Health Serv Res Policy* 1999; 4:204–209.

24. Rothschild JM. Ultrasound guidance of central vein catheterization. In: Shojania KG, Duncan BW, McDonald KM, et al., eds. *Making Health Care Safer: A Critical Analysis of Patient Safety Practices.* Evidence Report/Technology Assessment No. 43, AHRQ Publication No. 01-E058. Rockville, MD: Agency for Healthcare Research and Quality, July 2001.

25. Jones PW, Moyers JP, Rogers JT, et al. Ultrasound-guided thoracentesis: Is it a safer method? *Chest* 2003;123:418–423.

26. Garg AX, Adhikari NK, McDonald H, et al. Effects of computerized clinical decision support systems on practitioner performance and patient outcomes: a systematic review. *JAMA* 2005;293:1223–1238.

27. Berner ES, Webster GD, Shuerman AA, et al. Performance of four computer-based diagnostic systems. *N Engl J Med* 1994;330:1792–1796.

28. Ramnarayan P, Winrow A, Coren M, et al. Diagnostic omission errors in acute paediatric practice: impact of a reminder system on decision-making. *BMC Med Inform Decis Mak* 2006; 6:37.

29. Payne TH, Nichol WP, Hoey P, et al. Characteristics and override rates of order checks in a practitioner order entry system. *Proc AMIA Symp* 2002;2002:602–606.

30. Wachter RM. Expected and unanticipated consequences of the quality and information technology revolutions. *JAMA* 2006;295:2780–2783.

31. Poon EG, Blumenthal D, Jaggi T, et al. Overcoming barriers to adopting and implementing computerized physician order entry systems in U.S. hospitals. *Health Aff (Millwood)* 2004;23:184–190.

ADDITIONAL READINGS

Ash JS, Berg M, Coiera E. Some unintended consequences of information technology in health care: the nature of patient care information system-related errors. *J Am Med Inform Assoc* 2004;11:104–112.

Aspden P, Wolcott J, Bootman JL, et al., eds. *Preventing Medication Errors: Quality Chasm Series*. Committee on Identifying and Preventing Medication Errors. Washington, DC: National Academy Press, 2007.

Cochran GL, Jones KJ, Brockman J. Errors prevented by and associated with bar-code medication administration systems. *Jt Comm J Qual Patient Saf* 2007;33:293–301.

Cutler DM, Feldman NE, Horwitz JR. U.S. adoption of computerized physician order entry systems. *Health Aff (Millwood)* 2005;24:1654–1663.

Hunt DL, Haynes RB, Hanna SE, et al. Effects of computer-based clinical decision support systems on physician performance and patient outcomes: a systematic review. *JAMA* 1998;280:1339–1346.

Kuperman GJ, Gibson RF. Computerized physician order entry: benefits, costs, and issues. *Ann Intern Med* 2003;39:31–39.

Shekelle PG, Morton SC, Keeler EB. Costs and Benefits of Health Information Technology. Evidence Report/Technology Assessment No. 132 (Prepared by the Southern California Evidence-based Practice Center under Contract No. 290-02-0003. Rockville, MD: Agency for Healthcare Research and Quality, April 2006. AHRQ Publication No. 06-E006.)

CHAPTER FOURTEEN

Reporting Systems, Incident Investigations, and Other Methods of Understanding Safety Issues

OVERVIEW

As patients, reporters, and legislators began to appreciate the scope of the medical errors problem in the late 1990s, the response was nearly Pavlovian: we need more reporting! This commonsensical appeal to transparency assumes that simply making errors public will create sufficient incentives—everything from embarrassment to legislation—to drive improvements in safety.

Although this chapter will discuss reporting systems of all kinds, most reporting is local (i.e., within the walls of a hospital). The systems to capture local reports are generally known as *incident reporting* (IR) systems. Incident reports come from frontline personnel (e.g., the nurse, pharmacist, or physician caring for a patient when a medication error occurred) rather than, say, from supervisors. From the perspective of those collecting the data, IR

153

systems are *passive* forms of surveillance, relying on involved parties to choose to report. More *active* methods of surveillance, such as retrospective chart review, direct observation, and trigger tools, will be discussed later. Although IR systems capture only a fraction of incidents, they have the advantages of relatively low cost and the involvement of caregivers in the process of identifying important problems for the organization.

I believe that the following realities should frame discussions of the role of reporting in patient safety:

- Errors occur one at a time, to patients—often already quite ill— scattered through hospitals, nursing homes, and doctors' offices. This generates tremendous opportunity to cover up errors, and requires that providers be engaged in efforts to achieve transparency.

- Because reporting errors takes time and can lead to shame and—particularly in the United States—legal liability, providers need to be protected from unfair blame, public embarrassment, and legal risk.

- Reporting systems need to be easy to access and use, and reporting must yield palpable improvements. Because passive reporting systems depend on the voluntary actions of frontline personnel, busy caregivers are unlikely to report if systems are burdensome or they feel that their reports disappear into a bureaucracy.

- The need to learn from errors permeates the system and its stakeholders. Doctors, nurses, hospital administrators, educators, researchers, regulators, legislators, the media, and patients all have different levels of understanding and may need to see very different types of reports. This diversity makes error reporting particularly challenging.

- Although most errors do reflect systems problems, some can be attributed to bad providers. The public—and those chartered to defend the public's interest, such as licensing and credentialing boards—have a legitimate need to learn of these cases and take appropriate (including disciplinary) action.

- Similarly, even when the problem is systemic and not one of "bad apples," the public has a right to know about systems that are sufficiently unsafe that a reasonable person would hesitate before receiving care from them.

- Medical errors are so breathtakingly common that the admonition to "report everything" is silly. The average intensive care unit (ICU) patient has 1.7 errors in his or her care daily, and the average hospitalized patient experiences one medication error per day.[1] A system that captured every error and near miss would quickly accumulate unmanageable mountains of data, require an armada of analysts, and result in caregivers spending much of their time reporting instead of caring for patients.

Taken together, these "facts on the ground" mean that a strategy of reporting errors, while conceptually attractive, must be approached thoughtfully. IR systems must be easy to use, nonpunitive, and manned by people skilled at analyzing the data and putting it to use. Moreover, given the limitations of IR systems, other techniques should also be employed to capture errors and identify risky situations. This chapter will cover a few, including *failure mode and effects analysis* (FMEA) and *trigger tools*. Errors that are reported must be put to good use, often by turning them into stories that are shared within organizations, such as through *Morbidity and Mortality (M&M) conferences*. Finally, errors that are particularly concerning—known as *sentinel events*—must be analyzed in a way that rapidly generates the maximum amount of institutional learning and catalyzes the appropriate changes. The following sections discuss each of these issues.

REPORTING SYSTEMS

Error reports, whether filed on paper or through the Web, and whether routed to the hospital's safety officer or to a federal regulator, can be divided into three main categories: anonymous, confidential, and open. *Anonymous reports* are ones in which there is no identifying information asked of the reporter. Although they have the advantage of encouraging reports, anonymous systems have the disadvantage of preventing often-necessary follow-up questions from being answered. In a *confidential reporting system*, the identity of the reporter is known but shielded from authorities such as regulators and representatives of the legal system (except in cases of clear professional misconduct or criminal acts). Such systems tend to capture better data than anonymous systems, because follow-up questions can be asked. The key to these systems, of course, is that reporters must trust that they are truly confidential. Finally, in *open reporting systems* all people and places are publicly identified. These systems have a relatively poor track record in medicine, because the potential for unwanted publicity and blame is so strong, and it is usually easy

---

TABLE 14–1

Characteristics of an ideal reporting system

- All stakeholders on board
- Intent and goals clear to all parties
- "Just" culture: reporters protected as much as possible from legal and other harms
- Accountability issues clear, focused, understandable—limited to reckless intent and violation
- Reporting includes both confidential and anonymous options
- Anyone can report
- Reporting made as easy as possible; multiple options
- Narrative as well as fixed field, choice selection data collection forms
- Field experts used for data analysis
- Feedback to all stakeholders, especially reporters, is rapid cycle and relevant
- Sustained leadership critical to protect core mission and values

---

Reproduced with permission from http://www.ahrq.gov/about/cpcr/ptsafety/ambpts4.htm# Characteristics.

for individuals to cover up errors (even with "mandatory" reporting). The Agency for Healthcare Research and Quality has summarized the attributes of an effective reporting system (Table 14–1).

Another distinguishing feature of reporting systems is the organizational entity that receives the reports. With that in mind, we will first consider the local hospital system—the IR system—and then widen the lens to systems that move reports to other entities beyond the clinical organization's walls.

HOSPITAL INCIDENT REPORTING SYSTEMS

Hospitals have long had IR systems, but traditional systems relied on providers (nearly always nurses—most studies show that nurse reports outnumber physician reports by at least 5:1[2]) to fill out paper reports. The reports generally went to the hospital's risk manager, whose main concern was often to limit her institution's potential legal risk. There was little emphasis on systems improvement, and dissemination of incidents to others in the system (other managers, caregivers, educators) was unusual. Most clinicians felt that reporting was a waste of time, and so few did it.

Over the past decade, IR systems have improved in technology, oversight, and philosophy. Many hospitals have computerized systems, in which any provider can submit an incident and categorize it by error type (e.g., medication error, patient fall; Table 14–2) and level of harm (e.g., no harm, minimal harm, serious harm, death). In confidential systems, the reporter can be contacted to provide additional detail if needed. Computerized systems make it easy to create aggregate statistics about the reports, although it is

---

TABLE 14–2

Typical major categories in a hospital IR system

- Anesthesia issues
- Behavior management (including restraint use/seclusion)
- Cardiac and respiratory arrest
- Confidentiality and consent issues
- Controlled substance issues
- Diagnosis/treatment issues
- Dietary services
- Environmental safety
- Falls/injuries (patient)
- Home care issues
- Infection control (including bloodborne pathogens, isolation issues)
- IVs, tubes, catheter, and drain issues (including broken, infiltrated catheters)
- Laboratory results (including result errors, tests not performed, wrong specimens)
- Medical devices (including device malfunction, improper use)
- Medication-related events (including errors, delays, and adverse drug reactions)
- Patient flow issues
- Patient property loss
- Radiology issues
- Security issues
- Skin issues (including pressure ulcers)
- Surgical issues (including death in operating room, retained objects, unplanned return to OR)
- Sterile processing issues
- Skin issues
- Transfusion issues
- Unprofessional staff behavior

important to recognize that voluntary systems are incapable of providing accurate error "rates."[3] For example, the hospital whose monthly incidents spike from 70 to 100 may be less safe (more reported errors) or more safe (people are more willing to report, feeling that they will be treated appropriately and that their reports will result in meaningful action)—there is simply no way to know. Probably most importantly, the reports can be routed to the managers positioned to take action or spot trends (unfortunately, not all computerized IR systems have this functionality). For example, when an error pertaining to the medical service is reported through my hospital's computerized IR system, the system automatically sends an e-mail to me (as chief of the service) as well as the service's head nurse, the hospital's risk manager, the "category manager" (an appropriate individual is assigned to each item in Table 14–2), and the hospital's director of patient safety. We each review the error, often have a discussion about it (orally or via a list serve within the IR system), and take the appropriate action.

Although this represents great progress, it is important to appreciate the amount of time, skill, and energy all of these functions take. Many hospitals have built IR systems, proceeded to exhort their staff to "report everything—errors, near misses, everything," and then found themselves overwhelmed by thousands of reports. I'd much rather see a system that received fewer reports but that acted on the reports effectively, than one with larger numbers of reports that end up in the black hole of a hospital's hard drive.

REPORTS TO ENTITIES OUTSIDE THE HEALTHCARE ORGANIZATION

Things get even dicier when we move the reports beyond the walls of a hospital or clinic. At this writing, for example, more than half the states in the United States have implemented mandatory reporting programs, to which some hospital errors must be reported.[4] The State of Pennsylvania has a system that requires hospitals to report all "serious events," "incidents," and hospital-acquired infections. Similarly, the United Kingdom's National Patient Safety Agency (NPSA) has had a national reporting system for "patient safety incidents" since 2004. At this writing, Pennsylvania has collected 400,000 reports, while the United Kingdom has more than 1 million! Each entity is actively trying to figure out what to do with all these data.[5] This is not to say that there is no value—Pennsylvania, for example, puts out a quarterly newsletter that describes important errors and patterns gleaned from the reports. But it is an open question (one whose answer I am skeptical about) whether the value of state, or particularly federal, reporting systems will be worth the substantial resources they require. In another approach pioneered by Minnesota, a few states require that hospitals report errors that rise to the level of the National Quality Forum's "Never Events" (Appendix VI). In 2005–2006, 154 such errors were publicly reported (with the reporting hospitals identified) in Minnesota, a much more manageable number than Pennsylvania's hundreds of thousands.

The pressure to build statewide or federal reporting systems grew in part (like so much of the patient safety field) from the experience of commercial aviation. One question worth considering as we debate expanding reporting systems is whether this particular analogy is apt.

On December 1, 1974, a Trans World Airlines (TWA) flight crashed into the side of a small mountain in Virginia, killing all 92 passengers and crew. As tragic as the crash was, the subsequent investigation added insult to injury, because the problems leading to the crash were well known to many pilots (poorly defined minimum altitudes on the Dulles Airport approach) but not widely disseminated. A year later, the Federal Aviation Administration (FAA) launched the *Aviation Safety Reporting System* (ASRS). Importantly, recognizing that airline personnel might be hesitant to report errors and near misses to their primary regulator, FAA contracted with a third party (NASA) to run the system and disseminate its lessons.

The ASRS rules are straightforward and designed to encourage reporting and dissemination. First, if anyone witnesses a near miss (note an important different from healthcare: nonnear misses in aviation—i.e., hits—don't need a reporting system, because they appear on the news within minutes), they *must* report it to ASRS within 10 days. The reporter is initially identified so that he or she can be contacted, if needed, by ASRS personnel; the identifying information is subsequently destroyed. In 30 years of operation, there have been no reported confidentiality breaches of the system. Trained ASRS personnel analyze the reports for patterns, and they have a number of pathways to disseminate key information or trigger actions (including grounding airplanes if necessary). There is general agreement that the ASRS is one of the main reasons for aviation's remarkable safety record (a 10-fold decrease in fatalities over the past generation; Figure 9–1).

Five attributes of the ASRS have helped create these successes: ease of reporting, confidentiality, third-party administration, timely analysis and feedback, and the possibility of regulatory action. But even as health-care tries to emulate these successes, it is worth highlighting some major dissimilarities between its problems and those of commercial aviation. The biggest difference is the scale of the two enterprises and their errors.[6] Notwithstanding its extraordinary effort to encourage reporting, the ASRS receives about 30,000 reports per year.[7] If all errors and near misses were being reported in American healthcare, this would almost certainly result in more than 30,000 reports *per day*—over 10 million reports per year! The system is simply far more complex, with far more opportunities for things to go wrong, and so the issues of prioritizing and managing the reports are far knottier.

My personal belief is that mandatory, confidential reporting to a larger organization (either a national one such as the Joint Commission or state entities such as in Minnesota) is a reasonable idea for sentinel or "Never Events": errors that led to patient deaths or significant disability, or those that should "never happen" (Appendix VI). Assuming that this process was well managed and legally protected, such a system could ensure that any corrective action would be effective and could be enforced if necessary. I also believe that the reports should remain confidential, in order to encourage reporting (the exception being for egregious errors or those that illustrate a pattern of unsafe behavior). I fear that a system completely open to the public would lead to more cover-ups and further the environment of defensiveness.

ROOT CAUSE ANALYSIS AND OTHER INCIDENT INVESTIGATION METHODS

After we learn of a significant error, what do we do? The technique of *root cause analysis* (RCA) involves a deliberate, comprehensive dissection of an error, laying bare all of the relevant facts but searching assiduously for underlying ("root") causes rather than being satisfied by facile explanations (such as "the doctor pulled the wrong chart" or "the pharmacist stocked the wrong medicine"). To ensure that RCAs are maximally productive, certain elements appear to be important:

1. *Strong leadership and facilitation*: it is easy for a RCA to gravitate away from the search for root causes and toward the assignment of blame. The leader needs to be skilled at steering the conversation toward the key systems defects, including complex

and potentially charged issues involving culture and communication. The use of a structured tool to prompt participants to consider the full range of potential contributing factors can be helpful (Table 2–1).[8]

2. *An interdisciplinary approach*: the RCA committee should include representatives of all of the relevant disciplines (at a minimum, physicians, nurses, pharmacists, and administrators). In addition, a risk manager is often present, although the discussion should focus on what can be learned from the error rather than on how to reduce the institution's liability. In larger organizations, content experts (such as in information technology and human factors) can add insights.

3. *Individuals who participated in the case should be invited to "tell their stories."* These discussions can be highly emotional, and the RCA leader needs to skillfully manage the presentation of facts to ensure maximum benefit, paying particular attention to avoiding finger-pointing and subsequent defensiveness. It is often useful for someone (usually the patient safety officer or risk manager) to have gathered many of the key facts and timelines and present them to the RCA committee so that the discussion can focus on aspects of the case that cannot be ascertained from the medical record. However, even when this has been done, it is important to confirm the facts with the participants early in the meeting. In some cases, it is best to have all the involved caregivers present at the same meeting to share their views of the case; in others, this will be too emotionally charged and sequential presentations may be preferable.

4. *Some institutions routinely invite other frontline workers (such as an uninvolved nurse or physician) to RCAs* to help educate them in the process and demystify the ritual. The hope is that they can serve as ambassadors for the process with their colleagues. Other organizations have found that the participation of lay individuals adds an important perspective.

The goal of the RCA is to identify systems factors that led to the error, and to suggest solutions that can prevent similar errors from causing harm in the future.[8–10] However, in its zeal to emphasize systems factors, the RCA committee should not shy away from identifying human error, nor from taking appropriate steps to ensure accountability (such as when there is evidence of repetitive errors by a single individual or of failure to adhere to sensible safety rules) (Chapter 19). Often, these situations will create a need to take the findings to a more appropriate venue, such as a medical staff credentialing committee. As with many aspects of trying to improve patient safety, finding the appropriate balance between a systems approach and individual accountability is the most challenging aspect of the RCA process.

MORBIDITY AND MORTALITY CONFERENCES

While the RCA process is confidential, many institutions have recognized the value of presenting cases of medical errors to diverse groups of providers, usually in an *M&M conference*. Case of medical errors are often quite interesting and dramatic, and a well-constructed "M&M" can quickly become one of the premier educational sessions in an institution. As with the RCA, it is vital that the leader be a skilled facilitator— striving to protect the presenter (if he or she participated in the care of the patient) from public humiliation, and working to elucidate systems factors that bear improvement or general lessons for the audience. Although most M&M conferences involve physicians only and focus on a single discipline (i.e., surgery or medicine), innovations include interdisciplinary M&M conferences (e.g., with both physicians and nurses), cross-specialty M&M conferences (e.g., surgeons and internists), and conferences that involve institutional administrators and catalyze action and follow-up. In the latter model, after systems issues are uncovered in the conference, a group is charged with returning later to present what was learned about the issue and how it was fixed. One study demonstrated that internal medicine M&M conferences are often too reluctant to classify errors as errors (tending instead to divert into academic discussions of pathophysiology or more traditional aspects of diagnosis and therapy), while surgical conferences tend to focus unduly on individual fault at the cost of insufficient focus on systems issues.[11]

Unfortunately, many hospitals (particularly nonacademic ones) and departments lack M&M conferences, and they are rare in outpatient settings. Reasons cited include fear of medicolegal risk (although the content of M&M conferences is protected from legal exposure if they are performed under the hospital's quality assurance umbrella[12]), and the absence of time or expertise. Luckily, there are now several academic series that provide M&M-type analyses of errors, including several that I have been privileged to write or edit: the Quality Grand Rounds series in the *Annals of Internal Medicine* (Appendix I), a popular book that analyzes dramatic cases of errors,[13] and a federally sponsored online M&M conference (AHRQ WebM&M).[14]

OTHER METHODS OF CAPTURING SAFETY PROBLEMS

It is important to recognize that IR systems are only one of several methods to capture safety problems. Increasingly, methods to identify "systems safety" through certain measurable structures, processes, and outcomes (Donabedian's Triad, Chapter 3) have been developed that do not depend on voluntary reporting. For example, if stronger evidence emerges that computerized provider order entry (CPOE) is associated with improved medication safety, the presence of a well-functioning CPOE system might be a reasonable structural marker of an institution's safety (Chapter 13). Using observers or even hidden cameras to see whether providers are washing their hands or surgical teams are conducting effective "time outs" before first incision might allow the assessment of process measures for safety. Outcome measures are trickier in that they usually require case-mix adjustment to ensure apples-to-apples comparisons. But in areas in which patients are relatively stereotypical (e.g., ICU patients on mechanical ventilators), rates of certain complications (ventilator-associated pneumonias, Chapter 10) might be reasonable measures of safety. Finally, because we now understand that the presence of appropriate structures (such as CPOE) and processes (time outs, signing the site) can be undermined by poor culture, measuring safety culture may be another important marker of systems safety. A number of surveys have now been validated for this purpose,[15,16] and emerging evidence shows that poor culture is associated with poor safety, and that improving culture may be associated with fewer errors. The next chapter will explore ways of doing that.

The use of *trigger tools* is an increasingly popular method to identify certain kinds of errors, particularly medication errors. These tools rely on the fact that many medication errors leave predictable footprints, such as the need for an antidote or the worsening of a blood test result. With this in mind, common trigger tools include the use of the opiate antagonist naloxone (indicating a possible overdose of opiates) or an international normalized ratio (INR) of >4 (therapeutic INR is usually 2–3) in a patient on warfarin (indicating over-anticoagulation). A list of commonly used triggers is given in

Table 1–1 (Chapter 1). It is important to recognize that trigger tools are overly sensitive, and must be followed by another method (usually a detailed chart review) to truly determine whether there was an error or even an adverse event[17–19]).

Finally, the technique of *failure mode and effects analysis* (*FMEA*), borrowed from engineering, is being used in many healthcare institutions to identify active and latent threats to safety.[20] In a FMEA, the likelihood that a particular process will fail is combined with an estimate of the relative impact of that error to produce a "criticality index." This index allows one to prioritize specific processes as quality improvement targets. For instance, a FMEA of the medication dispensing process on a hospital ward might break down all steps from receipt of orders in the central pharmacy to filling automated dispensing machines by pharmacy technicians (Chapter 4). Each step would be assigned a probability of failure and an impact score, so that all steps could be ranked according to the product of these two numbers. Steps ranked at the top would be prioritized for error proofing. The strength of the FMEA technique is that it taps into the insights of both experts and frontline workers to prioritize hazards and create an agenda for improvement. Anecdotally, institutions are reporting that FMEAs are leading to useful insights not obtainable from other methods.[21–23] It should be noted that FMEA is only one of an alphabet soup (PSA, SLIM, HAZOP, and so on) of human reliability techniques.[24]

KEY POINTS

- Although it is natural to favor reporting as an important component of improving patient safety (through "transparency"), several factors (including the ubiquity of errors, the difficulty capturing errors without voluntary reporting, and the multiple perspectives and stakeholders) make error reporting quite challenging.

- The most common reporting systems are institutionally-based voluntary IR systems. Efforts are underway to migrate reports to extrainstitutional entities such as states, the federal government, and regulators, with mixed results.

- Significant errors should be deeply investigated through a RCA, seeking systems problems that merit improvement.

- Sharing stories of errors is an important part of improving safety. This is usually done through an institutional M&M conference, though there are now outside resources that carry out similar functions.

- Other methods to capture safety problems include identifying the lack of evidence-based safety structures, processes, and outcomes, and the use of trigger tools and FEMA.

REFERENCES

1. Donchin Y, Gopher D, Olin M, et al. A look into the nature and causes of human errors in the intensive care unit. *Crit Care Med* 1995;23:294–300.
2. Wild D, Bradley EH. The gap between nurses and residents in a community hospital's error-reporting system. *Jt Comm J Qual Patient Saf* 2005;31:13–20.
3. Pronovost PJ, Miller MR, Wachter RM. Tracking progress in patient safety: an elusive target. *JAMA* 2006;296:696–699.
4. Rosenthal J, Booth M. *Maximizing the Use of State Adverse Event Data to Improve Patient Safety.* Portland, ME: National Academy for State Health Policy, 2005.
5. In conversation with . . . Sir Liam Donaldson. AHRQ WebM&M (serial online), May 2006. Available at: http://webmm.ahrq.gov/perspective.aspx?perspectiveID=40
6. Wilf-Miron R, Lewenhoff I, Benvamini Z, et al. From aviation to medicine: applying concepts of aviation safety to risk management in ambulatory care. *Qual Saf Health Care* 2003;12:35–39.
7. Barach P, Small SD. Reporting and preventing medical mishaps: lessons from non-medical near miss reporting systems. *BMJ* 2000;320:759–763.
8. Bagian JP, Gosbee J, Lee CZ, et al. The Veterans Affairs root cause analysis system in action. *Jt Comm J Qual Improv* 2002;28:531–545.
9. Rex JH, Turnbull JE, Allen SJ, et al. Systematic root cause analysis of adverse drug events in a tertiary referral hospital. *Jt Comm J Qual Improv* 2000;26:563–575.
10. Chassin MR, Becher EC. The wrong patient. *Ann Intern Med* 2002; 136:826–833.
11. Pierluissi E, Fischer MA, Campbell AR, et al. Discussion of medical errors in morbidity and mortality conferences. *JAMA* 2003;290:2838–2842.
12. Stewart RM, Corneille MG, Johnston J, et al. Transparent and open discussion of errors does not increase malpractice risk in trauma patients. *Ann Surg* 2006;243:645–651.

13. Wachter RM, Shojania KG. *Internal Bleeding: The Truth Behind America's Terrifying Epidemic of Medical Mistakes*. New York, NY: Rugged Land, 2004.
14. Available at: http://webmm.ahrq.gov
15. Pronovost P, Sexton B. Assessing safety culture: guidelines and recommendations. *Qual Saf Health Care* 2005;14:231–233.
16. Colla JB, Bracken AC, Kinney LM, et al. Measuring patient safety climate: a review of surveys. *Qual Saf Health Care* 2005;14:364–366.
17. Rozich JD, Haraden CR, Resar RK. Adverse drug event trigger tool: a practical methodology for measuring medication related harm. *Qual Saf Health Care* 2003;12:194–200.
18. Resar RK, Rozich JD, Simmonds T, et al. A trigger tool to identify adverse events in the intensive care unit. *Jt Comm J Qual Patient Saf* 2006;32:585–590.
19. Szekendi MK, Sullivan C, Bobb A, et al. Active surveillance using electronic triggers to detect adverse events in hospitalized patients. *Qual Saf Health Care* 2006;15:184–190.
20. McDermott RE, Mikulak RJ, Beauregard MR. *The Basics of FMEA*. Portland, OR: Resources Engineering, Inc., 1996.
21. DeRosier J, Stalhandske E, Bagian JP, et al. Using health care failure mode and effect analysis: the VA National Center for Patient Safety's prospective risk analysis system. *Jt Comm J Qual Improv* 2002;28:248–267.
22. Linkin DR, Sausman C, Santos L, et al. Applicability of healthcare failure mode and effects analysis to healthcare epidemiology: evaluation of the sterilization and use of surgical instruments. *Clin Infect Dis* 2005; 41:1014–1019.
23. Bonnabry P, Cingria L, Ackermann M, et al. Use of a prospective risk analysis method to improve the safety of the cancer chemotherapy process. *Int J Qual Health Care* 2006;18:9–16.
24. Lyons M, Adams S, Woloshynowych M, et al. Human reliability analysis in healthcare: a review of techniques. *Int J Risk Safe Med* 2004;16:223–237.

ADDITIONAL READINGS

Introduction to Trigger Tools for Identifying Adverse Events. Institute for Healthcare Improvement. Available at: http://www.ihi.org/IHI/Topics/PatientSafety/SafetyGeneral/Tools/IntrotoTriggerToolsforIdentifyingAEs.htm.
Longo DR, Hewett JE, Ge B, et al. The long road to patient safety: a status report on patient safety systems. *JAMA* 2005; 294:2858–2865.

Olsen S, Neale G, Schwab K, et al. Hospital staff should use more than one method to detect adverse events and potential adverse events: incident reporting, pharmacist surveillance and local real-time record review may all have a place. *Qual Saf Health Care* 2007;16:40–44.

Wachter RM, Shojania KG. The faces of errors: a case-based approach to educating providers, policy makers, and the public about patient safety. *Jt Comm J Qual Saf* 2004;31:665–670.

Weissman JS, Annas CL, Epstein AM, et al. Error reporting and disclosure systems: views from hospital leaders. *JAMA* 2005; 293:1359–1366.

CHAPTER FIFTEEN

Creating a Culture of Safety

OVERVIEW

In Chapter 9, I discussed the tragic collision of two 747s on a foggy morning in Tenerife, the crash that vividly illustrated to commercial aviation the risks associated with steep and unyielding authority gradients. In response to Tenerife and other similar accidents, aviation began a series of training programs, generally called "Crew Resource Management" or "Cockpit Resource Management" (CRM) programs, designed to train diverse crews in communication and teamwork. Some of these programs also incorporate communication skills, such as training in SBAR (Situation, Background, Assessment, and Recommendations) techniques (Chapter 9).

As healthcare came to understand the contribution of poor culture, communication, and teamwork to medical errors, efforts have begun to create healthcare versions of CRM programs to help solve these problems. Because these programs are so new, there are few data available to prove that they truly improve safety; the emerging evidence is positive but mixed.[1-3] Part of the challenge in studying these programs is the wide variation in the way they are conducted. From the literature and my own experience, the following elements appear to be important:

1. *Employ strong leadership and "champions"*: Culture change is hard, and one person's "empowerment" might be another's "depowerment." The case for culture change has to be clearly articulated, and buy-in—particular from those atop the authority gradient (in most cases, senior physicians)—is vital. Luckily, thoughtful physicians are increasingly appreciating the safety

risks associated with poor teamwork and steep authority gradients, and many are embracing CRM-type programs.

2. *Use aviation or other relevant nonhealthcare analogies, but don't overdo them*: The Tenerife story and others like it are wonderful ways to energize a healthcare audience, and—particularly for physicians—the pilots' stories are quite relevant. Pilots can confess to medical audiences that their culture was previously similar to that of physicians, and that they participated in CRM-type programs reluctantly at first—but that they now have come to believe that such training is essential to improving culture and decreasing errors. However, healthcare providers will be quick to highlight the differences between an operating room and a cockpit, and so the examples should quickly shift to medical ones. (The biggest difference: the "team" in a cockpit is generally two or three individuals with similar training, expertise, income, and social status. Dampening this hierarchy is easy compared to doing so in a busy operating room or labor and delivery suite, where the gradient might span from the chief of neurosurgery or obstetrics to a ward clerk who is a recent immigrant with a high school degree; Chapter 9.)

3. *Consider whether to use simulation*: There is active debate regarding the utility of simulation in facilitating CRM-type culture and communication training (there is less debate on the utility of simulation for improving technical skills; Chapters 5 and 17).[4] Proponents of simulation in CRM training argue that it "raises the stakes," allows participants to suspend disbelief more readily, and makes lessons more memorable.[5] Others feel that simulation (particularly high fidelity, realistic simulation, as opposed to role-playing case scenarios) is not worth the added cost and complexity, and might even distract providers from the lessons regarding communication and collaboration.[6] Whether simulation is or is not used, it is critical to "get everybody in the room" to work through case-based scenarios, and to provide an opportunity for skillful debriefing and interdisciplinary cross talk.

4. *Programs must live on beyond the initial training*: Although a brief (e.g., 4–6 hours) CRM program can sensitize workers to some of the key cultural and communication issues, effective programs must outlive the initial training. For example, at the University of California, San Francisco (UCSF) we have established an interdisciplinary group of unit-based champions to run Morbidity and Mortality (M&M) conferences on the units, to serve as a

TABLE 15-1

Elements of the UCSF Crew Resource Management ("Triad for Optimal Patient Safety," TOPS) curriculum

Topic	Description	Time (min)
Welcome	From a system leader (i.e., chief medical officer)	10
"Laying the Foundation"	Brief overview, goals of the day	15
First, Do No Harm*	Video, then facilitated discussion to serve as icebreaker	40
Lecture on Healthcare Team Behaviors & Communication Skills	Delivered by a commercial airline pilot. Introduces key principles of safety culture, communication, inc. SBAR, CUS words (Chapter 9)	60
Small-group facilitated "scenarios"	Two case scenarios, groups of ~8 people (must be interdisciplinary) to teach and practice standardized communication, team behaviors	80

*Powerful video based on actual events from malpractice claim files of a perinatal mistake that results in a mother's death. Can be obtained from the Partnership for Patient Safety. Available at: http://www.p4ps.org/interactive_videos.asp.

The TOPS project was funded by the Gordon and Betty Moore Foundation.

sounding board for staff to present safety problems, and to engage in collective problem-solving. Such "unit-based safety teams" appear to be useful adjuncts to CRM-type training, especially when supported by a strong leadership commitment and appropriate tools[7,8] (see also Chapter 22).

A curricular for our CRM program at UCSF is shown in Table 15–1.

THE CULTURE OF LOW EXPECTATIONS

In a large teaching hospital, an elderly woman ("Joan Morris") is waiting to be discharged after a successful neurosurgical procedure. A floor away, another woman with a similar last name ("Jane Morrison") is scheduled to receive the day's first cardiac electrophysiology study (EPS), a procedure that starts and stops the heart repetitively to find the cause of a potentially fatal heart rhythm disturbance. The EPS laboratory calls the floor to send "Morrison" down, but the clerk hears "Morris" and tells that patient's nurse that the lab is ready for her patient. That's funny, she thinks, my patient was here for a neurosurgical procedure. Well, she assumes, one of the docs must have ordered the test and not told me. So she sends the patient down.

Later that morning, the neurosurgery resident enters Joan Morris's room to discharge his patient, and is shocked to learn that his patient is in the EPS laboratory. He sprints there, only to be told by the cardiologists that they are in the middle of a difficult part of the procedure and can't listen to his concerns. Assuming that his attending physician ordered the test without telling him, he returns to his work.

Luckily, the procedure, which was finally aborted when the neurosurgery attending came to discharge his patient and learned she was in the EPS laboratory, caused no lasting harm (in fact, the patient later told us, "I'm glad my heart checked out OK").

In their masterful discussion of this case[9] in our Quality Grand Rounds series on medical errors (Appendix I), Chassin and Becher coined the term "the culture of low expectations." In reflecting on the actions—or inactions—of the nurse and the resident, they wrote,

> We suspect that these physicians and nurses had become accustomed to poor communication and teamwork. A 'culture of low expectations' developed in which participants came to expect a norm of faulty and incomplete exchange of information [which led them to conclude] that these red flags signified not unusual, worrisome harbingers but rather mundane repetitions of the poor communication to which they had become inured.[9]

Fighting the culture of low expectations is one of the most important elements of creating a safety culture. Doing this requires a change in default setting of all the providers, from:

A. If you're not sure it is wrong, assume it is right (it's probably just another glitch, we have them all the time around here),

to

B. If you're not sure it's right, assume that it is wrong (and do whatever it takes to become sure, even if it delays the first case in the operating room or makes someone irritated).

There is no shortcut to fighting the culture of low expectations. Yes, it is important to clean up the communication (with tools like SBAR and CRM training; Chapter 9), so that the instinct to think, "another glitch, it must be right," becomes less automatic. But healthcare organizations will always have examples of faulty, ambiguous communication or rapid changes that cannot be communicated to everyone. Therefore, changing the mindset from default setting "A" to "B" requires a powerful and consistent message from senior leadership (Chapter 22). More importantly, when someone *does* take the time to perform a double check when something seems amiss—and it turns out everything was OK—it is vital for senior leaders to vocally and publicly support that person. If praise is bestowed for the true save but withheld for the clerk who stopped the presses but later learned that everything was as it should be, staff are unlikely to stick with mindset "B," because they will still fret about the negative consequences of being wrong.[10]

RAPID RESPONSE TEAMS

Analyses of deaths and unexpected cardiopulmonary arrests in hospitals have demonstrated that there are often signs of patient deterioration that go unnoticed for hours. Identifying these warning signs may require better technology (such as monitoring systems) or improved nurse staffing (Chapter 16). But the failure to intervene in these settings may also indicate a cultural problem: in some circumstances, root cause analyses demonstrate that a nurse appreciated something was awry and was either unable to find a physician or reluctant to bypass the traditional hierarchy (i.e., the standard procedure to call the private physician before the ICU physician, or the intern before the attending).

The concept of Rapid Response Teams (sometimes called "Medical Emergency Teams") was developed as a response to these problems. Now renamed "Rapid Response Systems" (RRS) to emphasize the importance of both the monitoring and the response,[11] such teams have been heavily promoted by some as a powerful patient safety intervention, and were included among the six "planks" of the Institute for Healthcare Improvement's "Campaign to Save 100,000 Lives" in 2005–2006 (Table 20–1). At this writing, the evidence supporting RRSs remains mixed,[12–14] although the concept has face validity. Whether RRSs become standard of care will depend on the evidence of their value, but the concept of empowering nurses (and others) to feel comfortable "breaking rank" to ensure patient safety is attractive.

OTHER METHODS TO PROMOTE CULTURE CHANGE

Achieving culture change is a leadership challenge, one that is intertwined with many of the other elements of an effective patient safety program. For example, Sexton has found that the question that most strongly predicts a positive safety culture on a unit is "I am encouraged by my colleagues to report any patient safety concerns I may have."[15] Obviously, a unit with strong, collaborative leadership, a reporting system that facilitates blameless reporting, and a tradition of acting on reports is likely to have a positive safety culture. Seeing senior leadership engaged in Executive Walk Rounds or an Adopt-a-Unit program (Chapter 22) can help cement a positive safety culture. Sexton's findings that safety culture tends to be unit-specific (i.e., the ICU might have superb safety culture while the step-down unit 50 yards away has poor culture; Chapter 9) illustrate that institutions can improve their culture by learning what works on better units and exporting those lessons to more problematic ones.[16]

Elsewhere, I have discussed other issues relating to culture, and I end the chapter with a few general reflections. Rather than emphasizing the issues above (teamwork and collaboration, dampening down authority gradients, fighting the culture of low expectations), some institutions define a safety culture in terms of the following questions:

- Do workers report errors?
- Is there a "no blame" culture?
- Is safety in the strategic plan?

As I've already discussed (Chapter 14), I don't believe that pushing workers to report, report, and report some more (particularly to an institutional or governmental reporting system) is likely to generate a safety culture. That said, local reporting (especially when there is a supportive unit leader who listens to problems and helps fix them, and when reports fuel engaging M&M conferences) seems to be quite important, and reporting can be a useful part of a broader effort to discover problems and engage frontline workers.

The issue of "no blame" is one of the most complex in the safety field. Throughout the book, I have discussed the importance of a systems approach, fighting the instinct to blame and replacing it with a focus on identifying system flaws that allow inevitable human error to cause harm.

That said, I believe that the "no blame" mantra has been taken by some to absurd levels. Blame *is* appropriate for individuals who make frequent, careless errors, for individuals who fail to keep up with their specialty or who come to work intoxicated, or for individuals who willfully fail to follow reasonable safety rules. Marx has promoted the concept of a *"Just Culture"* (rather than a "no blame" culture) as a way to reconcile an appropriate focus on "no blame" when caring, competent workers make errors, while holding individuals (and institutions) accountable for blameworthy errors or conditions. A Just Culture distinguishes between "human error" (inevitable, and managed through systems change), "at-risk behavior" (such as "workarounds"—managed by understanding and fixing the systems-related factors that promote such behaviors), and "reckless behavior" ("acting in conscious disregard of substantial and unjustifiable risk"), which is blameworthy and for which individuals should be held accountable. For example, the surgeon who refuses to sign his or her surgical site or participate in a time-out prior to surgery is engaging in reckless behavior, and should be disciplined.[17] Further discussions regarding accountability can be found in Chapter 19.

Finally, placing patient safety in, or even atop, an institution's strategic plan is no guarantee of a safe culture. Senior leadership and hospital boards make an important statement when they prioritize patient safety among their values and missions, but too many organizations and leaders offer lip service without promoting the effort and allocating the resources to make this commitment real.[18,19] Creating a safe culture is hard work. But once it is created, it is easy to identify its presence, and its absence.

KEY POINTS

- Creating a safety culture is hard work, and does not happen automatically.

- Many institutions are adapting aviation-style Crew Resource Management programs to healthcare, and early results of well-implemented programs are mixed but generally promising.

- One aspect of a safe culture is fighting "the culture of low expectations," in which workers assume faulty communication and therefore fail to perform double checks despite clear warning signs.

- Rapid Response Teams have been promoted as a way to bypass rigid hierarchies in order to ensure that deteriorating patients promptly receive the care they need.

- The concept of a "Just Culture" has been advanced to emphasize the importance of blending a systems focus with appropriate individual and institutional accountability.

REFERENCES

1. Morey JC, Simon R, Jay GD, et al. Error reduction and performance improvement in the emergency department through formal teamwork training: evaluation results of the MedTeams project. *Health Serv Res* 2002;37:1553–1581.
2. Salas E, Wilson KA, Burke CS, et al. Does crew resource management training work? An update, an extension, and some critical needs. *Hum Factors* 2006;48:392–412.
3. Nielsen PE, Goldman MB, Mann S, et al. Effects of teamwork training on adverse outcomes and process of care in labor and delivery: a randomized controlled trial. *Obstet Gynecol* 2007;109:48–55.
4. Shapiro MJ, Morey JC, Small SD, et al. Simulation based teamwork training for emergency department staff: does it improve clinical team performance when added to an existing didactic teamwork curriculum? *Qual Saf Health Care* 2004;13:417–421.
5. Gaba DM. What does simulation add to teamwork training? AHRQ WebM&M (serial online), March 2006. Available at: http://www.webmm.ahrq.gov/perspective.aspx?perspectiveID=20.
6. Pratt SD, Sachs BP. Team training: classroom training vs. high-fidelity simulation. AHRQ WebM&M (serial online), March 2006. Available at: http://www.webmm.ahrq.gov/perspective.aspx?perspectiveID=21.
7. Pronovost P, Weast B, Rosenstein B. Implementing and validating a comprehensive unit-based safety program. *J Patient Saf* 2005;1:33–40.
8. Pronovost P, King J, Holzmueller CG, et al. A web-based tool for the Comprehensive Unit-based Safety Program (CUSP). *J Comm J Qual Patient Saf* 2006;32:119–129.
9. Chassin MR, Becher EC. The wrong patient. *Ann Intern Med* 2002; 136:826–833.
10. Wachter RM. Low on the totem pole. AHRQ WebM&M (serial online), December 2005. Available at: http://webmm.ahrq.gov/case.aspx?caseID=110.
11. Devita MA, Bellomo R, Hillman K, et al. Findings of the first consensus conference on medical emergency teams. *Crit Care Med* 2006;34: 2463–2478.
12. Hillman K, Chen J, Cretikos M, et al. Introduction of the medical emergency team (MET) system: a cluster-randomised controlled trial. *Lancet* 2005;365:2091–2097.

13. Wachter RM, Pronovost PJ. The 100,000 lives campaign: a scientific and policy review. *Jt Comm J Qual Patient Saf* 2006;32:621–627.
14. Winters BD, Pham J, Pronovost PJ. Rapid response teams—walk, don't run. *JAMA* 2006;296:1645–1647.
15. In conversation with . . . J. Bryan Sexton. AHRQ WebM&M (serial online), December 2006. Available at: http://www.webmm.ahrq.gov/perspective. aspx?perspectiveID=34.
16. Huang DT, Clermont G, Sexton JB, et al. Perceptions of safety culture vary across the intensive care units of a single institution. *Crit Care Med* 2007; 35:165–176.
17. Marx D. Patient safety and the "just culture": a primer for health care executives. April 17, 2001. Available at: www.mers-tm.net/support/marx_ primer.pdf.
18. Gosfield AG, Reinertsen JL. The 100,000 lives campaign: crystallizing standards of care for hospitals. *Health Aff (Millwood)* 2005;24: 1560–1570.
19. Joshi MS, Hines SC. Getting the board on board: engaging hospital boards in quality and patient safety. *Jt Comm J Qual Patient Saf* 2006;32: 179–187.

ADDITIONAL READINGS

Donaldson L. *An Organisation with a Memory: Report of an Expert Group on Learning from Adverse Events in the NHS Chaired by the Chief Medical Officer.* London: The Stationery Office, 2000.

Kotter JP. Leading change: why transformation efforts fail. *Harv Bus Rev* 1995;73:59–67.

Pronovost PJ, Weast B, Holzmueller CG, et al. Evaluation of the culture of safety: survey of clinicians and managers in an academic medical center. *Qual Saf Health Care* 2003;12:405–410.

Vaughan D. *The Challenger Launch Decision: Risky Technology, Culture, and Deviance at NASA.* Chicago, IL: University of Chicago Press, 1997.

Weick KE, Sutcliffe KM. *Managing the Unexpected: Assuring High Performance in an Age of Complexity.* San Francisco, CA: Jossey-Bass, 2001.

CHAPTER SIXTEEN

Workforce Issues

OVERVIEW

In many discussions of patient safety, it is assumed that the workforce is up to the task: in training, competency, and numbers. In these formulations, a combination of the right processes, information technology, and culture are the ingredients for safe care.

However, as any frontline worker can tell you, neglecting issues of workforce sufficiency and competency omits an important part of the equation. For example, a nursing or physician workforce that is stretched and demoralized will result in unsafe conditions, even if the workers have good communication, rules, and computers. In this chapter, I will discuss some key issues in workforce composition and organizational structure. In the next chapter, I'll discuss issues of training and competency.

NURSING WORKFORCE ISSUES

Much of our understanding of the interaction between workforce and patient outcomes and medical errors relates to nursing. The combination of pioneering research,[1-4] a nursing shortage in the United States, and effective advocacy by nursing organizations (because most hospital nurses are salaried and employed by the hospitals, they have a strong incentive to advocate for sensible workloads; contrast this to physicians, most of whom are self-employed in the United States and therefore calibrate their own workload) has created this focus.

According to the American Hospital Association, demand for nurses now exceeds supply by 126,000; and one in seven U.S. hospitals report nursing vacancy rates of over 20%.[5] Because one-third of all U.S. nurses are over age 50, there will be more nurses leaving the profession than entering it by 2020, leaving a shortfall of about a million nurses to care for America's aging Baby Boomer generation, and even more stress for the remaining nurses. A 2002 American Hospital Association report high-lighted the problem: "Today, many in direct patient care feel tired and burned-out from a stressful, often understaffed environment, with little or no time to experience the one-on-one caring that should be the heart of hospital employment."[6]

Substantial data suggest that medical errors increase with higher ratios of patients to nurses. One study found that surgical patients had a 31% greater chance of dying in hospitals when the average nurse cared for more than seven patients. For every additional patient added to a nurse's average workload, patient mortality rose 7%, and nursing burnout and dissatisfaction increased 23% and 15%, respectively. The authors estimated that 20,000 annual deaths in the United States could be attrib-uted to inadequate nurse-to-patient ratios.[1] Regulators are beginning to consider adequacy of nurse staffing in their institutional assessments, and several states (including California) have legislated minimum nurse-to-patient ratios (usually 1:5 on medical-surgical wards and 1:2 in inten-sive care units). The jury is still out on whether these regulatory or legislative solutions are enhancing safety; some nurses note that ancillary personnel (clerks, lifting teams) have been released in order to hire enough nurses to meet the ratios, resulting in little additional time for nurses to perform nursing-related tasks.

Although some of the answers—better pay, benefits, and working conditions—to the nursing shortage will come through the traditional magic of competitive bargaining, new technology could play an impor-tant role as well, particularly if it relieves nurses of some of their paper-work burden and allows them to spend more time with their patients. In Chapter 13, I described the lunacy that results when a nurse takes a digital blood pressure reading and then wastes precious time in an error-prone struggle to transcribe it in multiple places. Situations like this, which go on dozens of times during a typical shift, are one reason many nurses believe so much of their time and training are wasted.

Importantly, even as the nursing shortage has catalyzed efforts to improve pay, hours, and technology, it has also brought overdue attention to issues of nursing culture and satisfaction. Unfortunately, studies in this area often point to problematic relationships with physician colleagues. In one survey of more than 700 nurses, 96% said they had witnessed or experienced disruptive behavior by physicians. Nearly half pointed to "fear of retribution" as the primary reason that such acts were not reported to superiors. Thirty percent of the nurses also said they knew at least one nurse who had resigned as a result of boorish—or worse—physician behavior, while many others knew nurses who had changed shifts or clinical units to avoid contact with particular offensive doctors.[7,8] These concern have been an important driver for the interdisciplinary training discussed in Chapter 15, and for increasing efforts to enforce acceptable standards of behavior among all healthcare professionals[9] (Chapter 19).

HOUSESTAFF DUTY HOURS

Amazingly, there is virtually no research linking safety or patient outcomes to the workload of practicing physicians. Dr. Michael DeBakey, the legendary Texas heart surgeon, was once said to have performed 18 cardiac bypass operations in a single day! The outcomes of the patients (particularly patient number 18) have not been reported. But the implicit message of such celebrated feats of endurance is that "real doctors" do not complain about their workload, they simply soldier on. With little research to rebut this attitude and with the dominant payment system in the United States rewarding productivity over safety, there have been few counterarguments to this machismo logic.

The one area in which this has changed is in the workload of physician trainees, particularly residents. At the core of residency training is being "on call"—staying in the hospital overnight to care for sick patients. Bad as things are now, they have markedly improved since the mid-1900s, when many residents actually *lived* at the hospital (giving us the term "house officer") for months at a time. Even as recently as 20 years ago, some residents were on call every other night, accumulating as many as 120 weekly work hours—which is particularly impressive when one considers that there are only 168 hours in a week!

Although resident call schedules have become somewhat more reasonable, many residents continued to be on call every third night, with over 100-hour workweeks, until very recently. But change has not come easily. As efforts to limit housestaff shifts gained momentum, some physician leaders argued that such hours were necessary to mint competent, committed physicians. For example, the editor of the *New England Journal of Medicine* wrote that long hours

. . . have come with a cost, but they have allowed trainees to learn how the disease process modifies patients' lives and how they cope with illness. Long hours have also taught a central professional lesson about personal responsibility to one's patients, above and beyond work schedules and personal plans. Whether this method arose by design or was the fortuitous byproduct of an arduous training program designed primarily for economic reasons is not the point. Limits on hours on call will disrupt one of the ways we've taught young physicians these critical values . . . We risk exchanging our sleep-deprived healers for a cadre of wide-awake technicians.[10]

Therein lies the tension: legitimate concerns that medical professionalism might be degraded by "shift work" and that excellence requires lots of practice and the ability to follow many patients from clinical presentation through work-up to denouement, balanced against concerns about the effects of fatigue on performance and morale.[11–13] The latter concerns are real. One study showed that 24 hours of sustained wakefulness results in performance equivalent to that of a person with a blood alcohol level of 0.1%—legally drunk in every state in the United States.[14] Although early researchers felt that this kind of impairment occurred only after very long shifts, we now know that chronic sleep deprivation is just as harmful. Healthy volunteers performing math calculations were just as impaired after sleeping 5 hours per night for a week as they were after a single 24-hour wakefulness marathon.[15] The investigators in this study didn't check to see what happened when both these disruptions occurred in the *same* week, the norm for many residents.

Although it defies common sense to believe that sleep-deprived brains and bad medical decisions are not related, hard proof of this intuitive link has been surprisingly hard to come by. Most studies using surgical simulators or videotapes of surgeons during procedures show that sleep-deprived residents have problems both with precision and efficiency, yet studies of nonsurgical trainees are less conclusive. One showed that interns who averaged less than 2 hours of sleep in the previous 32 hours made nearly twice as many errors reading ECGs, and had to give the tracings more attention, especially when reading several in a row. On the other hand, other studies showed that tired radiology residents made no more mistakes reading x-rays than well-rested ones, and sleepy ER residents performed physical examinations and recorded patient histories with equal reliability in both tired and rested conditions.[16,17]

In July 2003, the Accreditation Council for Graduate Medical Education (ACGME, the group that blesses the 7800 residency programs in the United States, involving over 100,000 trainees) stepped into the breech, limiting residents to a maximum of 80 hours per week, with no shift lasting longer than 30 consecutive hours and at least 1 day off per week (Table 16–1). Although the regulations seem like a reasonable beginning, there are surprisingly few data to prove that they will improve patient safety. In fact, a study of the impact of similar duty hours reductions instituted years earlier in New York State after the death of the daughter of a prominent reporter at a New York teaching hospital found that the number of hospital complications actually *went up*,[18,19] possibly because of the detrimental impact of additional handoffs (Chapter 8). A more recent study, however, did hint at a mortality benefit for medical patients after the ACGME regulations were enacted.[20]

In any case, the 80-hour limits have been implemented, and the debate continues. One study in the intensive care units of an academic medical center found that interns committed five times more serious diagnostic errors when working traditional 24- to 30-hour shifts than when their shifts were limited to an average of 15 hours.[21] A 2007 study showed that as the number of admissions per on-call resident increased, so did patient length of stay, costs, and mortality rate.[22] As stronger data emerge regarding the harmful effects of long shifts (including the now-legal

---

TABLE 16–1

Key elements of the ACGME's duty hours reduction policy

- An 80-h weekly limit, averaged over 4 weeks
- An adequate rest period, which should consist of 10 h of rest between duty periods
- A 24-h limit on continuous duty and up to 6 added hours for continuity of care and didactics
- One day in 7 free from patient care and educational obligations, averaged over 4 weeks
- In-house call no more than once every 3 nights, averaged over 4 weeks
- An option for programs in some specialties to request an increase of up to 8 h in weekly hours, with an educational rationale and approval of the sponsoring institution and relevant Residency Review Committee.

Reproduced with permission from http://www.acgme.org/acWebsite/dutyHours/dh_achieve Sum05-06.pdf.

30-hour shifts), further restrictions on resident duty hours seem likely. In fact, most other developed countries have far more stringent limits than those in the United States (Table 16–2). This continued shrinkage of duty hours will present a considerable challenge, since even today's 80-hour limits are routinely violated.[23]

In discussions regarding duty hours and fatigue, analogies are often made to other industries that have much more severe limits on consecutive work hours. For example, U.S. commercial pilots cannot fly for more than 8 hours straight without relief, and truck drivers must pull off the road after 10 hours for a mandatory break. But between these shifts, the machines either sit idle or are operated by another crew. Fumbles may occur in the handoffs of the machines but they are unusual, and no one hands over the reins in the middle of a critical function (like a airport landing approach). In medicine, on the other hand, handoff errors are dangerously routine (Chapter 8). This means that the real patient safety question is not whether fatigued doctors make more mistakes (they almost certainly do), but whether the errors caused by fumbled handoffs and more subtle information seepage will exceed those caused by fatigue.

However this equation is solved, there can be little debate on one issue: 100-hour workweeks *must* be bad for young doctors (and older

TABLE 16–2		
Housestaff work hours regulations in selected countries outside the United States		
	Maximum Hours/Week	**Maximum Hours/Shift**
United Kingdom	56, averaged	8–12
The Netherlands	48, averaged	10
Denmark	Not regulated, but average = 45	8–11
France	Not regulated; average = 50 plus on-call hours	No restrictions
Germany	56 h, averaged over 24 weeks	10
Australia	68–75	N/A

Reproduced with permission from Kwan R, Levy R. *A Primer on Resident Work Hours*. Reston, VA: American Medical Student Association, 2005. Available at: http://www.amsa.org/rwh/RWH-primer_6thEdition.pdf.

ones too, although no one is regulating their hours presently), their loved ones, and ultimately their patients. But regulations to limit duty hours must be accompanied by research to assess both the benefits and the risks of the limits and by aggressive programs to improve information transfer. At the University of California, San Francisco (UCSF), the duty hours regulations led us to develop standard procedures for patient handoffs (now required by the Joint Commission) and a robust information system module to promote safe handoffs (Figure 8.3).

In the end, something will undoubtedly be lost with the imposition of the new duty hours regulations. Whether that loss will be compensated for by parallel gains in safety remains to be seen. We may well see an increase in handoff fumbles, reduced educational time, and increased costs (as teaching hospitals are forced to replace relatively cheap housestaff labor with physicians assistants, nurse practitioners, or hospitalists). We may even see physicians' culture change from a "do whatever it takes" mindset to a "shiftwork" mentality, although residents remain quite torn by their understandable desire for more rest and their deeply felt ethical commitment to their patients.[24] All of these concerns can be mitigated somewhat by active efforts to make handoffs safer, to relieve residents of superfluous paperwork, to provide decent rest facilities in hospitals, and to compensate alternate providers to pick up the slack.

KEY POINTS

- Increasing attention is being paid to the importance of a well-trained, well-rested workforce to patient safety.

- In nursing, good studies have linked longer work hours and lower nurse-to-patient ratios to poor outcomes. This has led reform efforts, including legislation in some states.

- Although emerging research links long hours and fatigue in physicians to errors, it has not yet led to widespread efforts to regulate physician staffing. The exception is in residency programs, where regulations now limit duty hours.

- Duty hours limits must be accompanied by efforts to improve handoffs, lest the safety gains from less fatigue be lost through poor transitions of care.

REFERENCES

1. Aiken LH, Clarke SP, Sloane DM, et al. Hospital nurse staffing and patient mortality, nurse burnout, and job dissatisfaction. *JAMA* 2002; 288: 1987–1993.
2. Aiken LH, Clarke SP, Cheung RB, et al. Educational levels of hospital nurses and surgical patient mortality. *JAMA* 2003;290:1617–1623.
3. Rogers AE, Hwang WT, Scott LD, et al. The working hours of hospital staff nurses and patient safety. *Health Aff (Millwood)* 2004;23:202–212.
4. Hugonnet S, Chevrolet JC, Pittet D. The effect of workload on infection risk in critically ill patients. *Crit Care Med* 2007;35:76–81.
5. Steinbrook R. Nursing in the crossfire. *N Engl J Med* 2002;346:1757–1766.
6. AHA Commission on Workforce for Hospitals and Health Systems. *In Our Hands: How Hospital Leaders can Build a Thriving Workforce.* Chicago, IL: American Hospital Association, 2002.
7. Rosenstein AH, O'Daniel M. Disruptive behavior and clinical outcomes: perceptions of nurses and physicians. *Am J Nurs* 2005;105:54–64, quiz 64–65.
8. Rosenstein AH, O'Daniel M. Impact and implications of disruptive behavior in the perioperative arena. *J Am Coll Surg* 2006;203:96–105.
9. Leape LL, Fromson JA. Problem doctors: is there a system-level solution? *Ann Intern Med* 2006;144:107–115.
10. Drazen JM, Epstein AM. Rethinking medical training—the critical work ahead. *N Engl J Med* 2002;347:1271–1272.
11. Goitein L, Shanafelt TD, Wipf JE, et al. The effects of work-hour limitations on resident well-being, patient care, and education in an internal medicine residency program. *Arch Intern Med* 2005;165:2601–2606.
12. Lockley SW, Landrigan CP, Barger LK, et al. Harvard Work Hours Health and Safety Group. When policy meets physiology: the challenge of reducing resident work hours. *Clin Orthop Relat Res* 2006;449:116–127.
13. Hutter MM, Kellogg KC, Ferguson CM, et al. The impact of the 80-hour resident workweek on surgical residents and attending surgeons. *Ann Surg* 2006;243:864–871; discussion 871–875.
14. Dawson D, Reid K. Fatigue, alcohol and performance impairment. *Nature* 1997;388:235.
15. Linde L, Bergstrom M. The effect of one night without sleep on problem-solving and immediate recall. *Psychol Res* 1992;54:127–136.
16. Gaba DM, Howard SK. Patient safety: fatigue among clinicians and the safety of patients. *N Engl J Med* 2002;347:1249–1255.
17. Veasey S, Rosen R, Barzansky B, et al. Sleep loss and fatigue in residency training: a reappraisal. *JAMA* 2002;288:1116–1124.

18. Laine C, Goldman L, Soukup JR, et al. The impact of a regulation restricting medical house staff working hours on the quality of patient care. *JAMA* 1993;269:374–378.
19. Asch DA, Parker RM. The Libby Zion case. One step forward or two steps backward? *N Engl J Med* 1988;318:771–775.
20. Shetty KD, Bhattacharya J. Changes in hospital mortality associated with residency work-hour regulations. *Ann Intern Med* 2007;147:73–80.
21. Landrigan CP, Rothschild JM, Cronin JW, et al. Effect of reducing interns' work hours on serious medical errors in intensive care units. *N Engl J Med* 2004;351:1838–1848.
22. Ong M, Bostrom A, Vidyarthi A, et al. House staff team workload and organization effects on patient outcomes in an academic general internal medicine inpatient service. *Arch Intern Med* 2007;167:47–52.
23. Landrigan CP, Barger LK, Cade BE, et al. Interns' compliance with Accreditation Council for Graduate Medical Education work-hour limits. *JAMA* 2006;296:1063–1070.
24. Carpenter RO, Spooner J, Arbogast PG, et al. Work hours restrictions as an ethical dilemma for residents: a descriptive survey of violation types and frequency. *Curr Surg* 2006;63:448–455.

ADDITIONAL READINGS

Page A, ed. *Keeping Patients Safe: Transforming the Work Environment of Nurses.* Committee on the Work Environment for Nurses and Patient Safety, Board on Health Care Services. Washington, DC: National Academy Press, 2004.

Fletcher KE, Underwood W 3rd, Davis SQ, et al. Effects of work hour reduction on residents' lives: a systematic review. *JAMA* 2005;294:1088–1100.

Needleman J, Buerhaus P, Mattke S, et al. Nurse-staffing levels and the quality of care in hospitals. *N Engl J Med* 2002;346:1715–1722.

Needleman J, Buerhaus PI, Stewart M, et al. Nurse staffing in hospitals: is there a business case for quality? *Health Aff (Millwood)* 2006;25:204–211.

Vidyarthi AR, Auerbach AD, Wachter RM, et al. The impact of duty hours on resident self reports of errors. *J Gen Intern Med* 2007;22:205–209.

Weissman JS, Rothschild JM, Bendavid E, et al. Hospital workload and adverse events. *Med Care* 2007;45:448-455.

Wylie CD. Sleep, science, and policy change. *N Engl J Med* 2005;352:196–197.

CHAPTER SEVENTEEN

Training Issues

OVERVIEW

Medicine has a unique problem when it comes to its trainees. Although all fields must allow trainees some opportunity to "practice" their craft before being granted a credential allowing them to work without supervision, legal, accounting, or architectural errors made by trainees are generally less consequential than medical errors.

Moreover, the demands of medical practice (particularly the need for around-the-clock and weekend coverage) have led to the use of trainees as cheap labor, placing them in situations in which they have too little supervision for their skill level and experience. Although this early independence has been justified pedagogically as the need to allow "trainees to learn from their mistakes" and hone their clinical instincts, in truth much of it flowed from economic imperatives.

Yet the solution is not obvious. One can envision a training environment in which patients are protected from trainees—after all, who would not want the senior surgeon, rather than the second year resident, performing his cholecystectomy? While such an environment might be safer initially, the inevitable result would be more poorly trained physicians (and nurses and other caregivers) who lack the real world, supervised experience needed to transform them from novices into experienced professionals.

These two fundamental tensions form the backdrop of any discussion of training issues in the context of patient safety. First, what is the appropriate balance between autonomy and supervision? Second, are there ways for trainees to traverse their learning curves more quickly without necessarily "learning from their mistakes" on real patients? Other important training-related issues, such the importance of teamwork training in creating a safety culture and duty hour reductions for residents, are covered elsewhere in the book (Chapters 15 and 16, respectively).

AUTONOMY VERSUS OVERSIGHT

The third year medical student was sent in to "preround" on a patient, a 71-year-old man who had had a hip replacement a few days earlier. The patient complained of new shortness of breath, and on exam was anxious and perspiring, with rapid, shallow respirations. The student, on his first clinical rotation, listened to the man's lungs, expecting to hear the crackles of pulmonary edema or pneumonia or perhaps the wheezes of asthma, yet they were clear as a bell. The student was confused, and asked the patient what he thought was going on. "It's really hot in here, doc," said the patient, and, in fact, it was. The student reassured himself that the patient was just overheated, and resolved to discuss the case later that morning with his supervising resident. In his mind, calling the resident now would be both embarrassing and unnecessary—he had a good explanation for the patient's condition. An hour later, the patient was dead of a massive pulmonary embolism. The student never told anyone of his observations that morning, and felt shame about the case for decades afterwards.

In his wonderful book, *Complications,* Harvard surgeon Atul Gawande describes the fundamental paradox of medical training:

In medicine, we have long faced a conflict between the imperative to give patients the best possible care and the need to provide novices with experience. Residencies attempt to mitigate potential harm through supervision and graduated responsibility . . . . But there is still no getting around those first few unsteady times a young physician tries to put in a central line, remove a breast cancer, or sew together two segments of colon. No matter how many protections we put in place, on average, these cases go less well with the novice than with someone experienced.

This is the uncomfortable truth about teaching. By traditional ethics and public insistence (not to mention court rulings), a patient's right to the best care possible must trump the objective of training novices. We want perfection without practice. Yet everyone is harmed if no one is trained for the future. So learning is hidden behind drapes and anesthesia and the elisions of language.[1]

Traditionally, supervisors in medicine erred on the side of autonomy, feeling that trainees needed to learn by doing—giving rise to the iconic (but unethical) mantra of medical training, "see one, do one, teach one." We now recognize this paradigm as one more slice of the proverbial Swiss cheese, a constant threat to patient safety (Chapter 2).

Supervising physicians (the issues also play out with other health professionals such as nurses, but the autonomy that trainees in other fields can exercise and the danger they can cause are less than that of physicians) are terribly conflicted about all this. Supervisors know that they could do many things better and more safely, but also recognize that trainees truly do need to learn by doing. Moreover, providing the degree of supervision necessary to ensure that trainees never get into trouble would create job descriptions for supervising attendings (including around-the-clock presence) that might not be compatible with career longevity.

On a scale that has supervising physicians doing everything while the trainees watch at one pole, and trainees doing everything and calling their supervisors only when they are in trouble at the other, most medical training systems were far too tilted toward autonomy until fairly recently. Prodded by some widely publicized cases of medical error that were due, at least in part, to inadequate supervision (the death of Libby Zion at New York Hospital in 1986 was the most vivid example[2]; Table 1–1), the traditional model of medical education—dominated by unfettered resident autonomy—is giving way to something better. We now recognize that "learning from mistakes" is fundamentally unethical when it is built into the system, and that it is unreasonable to assume trainees will even know when they need help, particularly if they are thrust into the clinical arena with little or no practice and supervision.[3]

These recognitions have led not only to some system reforms, but also to a crack in the dike of academic medical culture. For example, many attendings now stay late with their teams on admitting nights, a practice that would have been judged pathologically obsessive only 20 years ago. In addition, the old culture of the "strong resident" or "strong student" (translated: one who never bothers his supervisors) is changing. Programs are increasingly building in expectations of oversight and creating structures to support it, such as around-the-clock attending presence (often hospitalists and intensivists) to help supervise trainees at night. They are also working with their trainees to make clear that a call for help and supervision is a sign of strength and professionalism, not weakness.

The challenge going forward will be to find the very narrow sweet spot between unfettered trainee autonomy and stifling attending oversight.[4]

Thankfully, driven in part by the patient safety movement, we are now much closer to this spot than we were even a decade ago.

By the way, I was the third year medical student who missed the fatal pulmonary embolism.[5]

THE ROLE OF SIMULATION

Although many discussions about medical simulation emphasize the ability of simulators to create realistic situations in which participants "suspend disbelief" (allowing for role plays that focus on teamwork and communication skills; Chapter 15), another key use of simulation is to allow individuals to traverse their procedural learning curves without harming patients. Even if we tested for procedural aptitude, like the military, novices' first few operations or procedures would still be hazardous to patients' health. Recognizing this, new surgeons traditionally work under the close supervision of a veteran—but not for very long. The old academic adage of "see one, do one, teach one" is fairly close to the mark in real life: after a couple of years of training, apprentice surgeons are largely on their own for all but the most complex cases.

The problem does not end once formal training is completed. After the completion of residency or fellowship, practicing surgeons and other interventionalists are essentially left on their own to acquire new skills or keep up with the latest techniques. In *Complications*, Gawande, himself a newly minted surgeon, writes that his father, a senior urologist in private practice, estimated that three-quarters of the procedures he now performs routinely did not exist when he was trained.[1] This means the issue of acquiring new skills safely is a lifelong challenge, not simply a training program issue.

Consider the case of laparoscopic gallbladder removal, "lap choley" for short. Since being introduced two decades ago, this technique has almost entirely replaced the much more invasive, and far more costly and risky "open choley." Laparoscopic techniques have also revolutionized other surgeries, including joint repair, hysterectomy, splenectomy, and even some open-heart surgeries.

The problem is that few surgeons trained before 1990 learned laparoscopic technique during their supervised apprenticeship. Is that a problem? Well, yes. One early study of lap choleys showed that injuries to the common bile duct dropped almost 20-fold once surgeons had performed more than 12 cases. And the learning curve continued: the rate of common bile duct injury on the 30th case was still 10 times higher than the rate seen after 50 cases.[6]

Until recently, the requirement that a surgeon certify his or her competency in any new procedure was nil—the system "trusted" that professionalism would ensure adequate training before physicians began practicing on patients, and there were few training models in which surgeons or other operators could efficiently learn new techniques without putting patients at risk. We spoke earlier (Chapters 8, 9, and 15) about what healthcare can learn from aviation when it comes to teamwork and communication. Here is yet another area in which aviation's approach to this problem—how to achieve competency, as quickly as possible, in high-risk situations using new equipment and procedures—seems far safer than medicine's.

In both commercial and military aviation, pilots prepare to fly new planes by first undergoing considerable formal training (in classrooms and in highly realistic simulators), followed by extensive, hands-on experience in the real thing, with an instructor pilot manning a dual set of controls seated next to the pilot. After that, pilots must pass both written and flight tests to qualify in the new machine, and they are continually evaluated with annual "check rides" administered by senior instructors. If a pilot flunks a check ride, he or she is put back on training status until the deficiencies are eradicated. When pilots fail several of these checks or are involved in a serious incident or accident, they are evaluated by what the Air Force calls a "Flight Evaluation Board," which has the power to clip their wings.

Contrast this with medicine's laissez-faire attitude toward recertification. Until relatively recently, there was no requirement for recertification in any specialty in American medicine, no requirement for demonstrated competency in new procedures, and no formal, required apprenticeship in new techniques (although some individual hospital medical staffs have enforced more rigorous criteria, and most states require some form of continuing education). This situation has improved in recent years: all major specialty boards now require recertification ("Maintenance of Certification" [MOC]) (Table 17–1) and a number of specialty societies have set minimum volume thresholds before allowing independent practice. And accrediting bodies (including the Accreditation Council for Graduate Medical Education and the Joint Commission) are enforcing more stringent requirements for competency-based credentialing of trainees and practicing physicians, respectively.

Even before these more rigorous requirements were enacted, many physicians *did* receive some training before beginning new procedures, driven by both individual professional integrity and the malpractice system.

	TABLE 17–1	
MOC requirements in key medical specialties in the United States		
Specialty	**No. of Years after First Board Certification before Recertification Required**	**Year That Recertification Became Mandatory**
Anesthesiology	10	2000
Emergency medicine	10	1980
Family practice	7	1970
Internal medicine	10	1990
Obstetrics and gynecology	6–10	1986
Diagnostic radiology	10	2002
Surgery	10	1995

But the data are sobering: a 1991 survey found that 55% of 165 practicing surgeons who had participated in a 2-day practical course on laparoscopic cholecystectomy felt the workshop had left them inadequately trained to start performing the procedure. Yet 74% of these surgeons admitted that they began performing lap choleys immediately after completing the course[7] (Chapter 5).

Now that the patient safety movement has convinced most observers that "learning on patients" is unethical when there are practical, safer alternatives, healthcare is increasingly looking to simulation. Procedural simulators have been around for decades in other industries. Military fliers used them even before World War II, although these "Link Trainers" were only crude approximations of the real thing. Static aircraft simulators (in which the cockpit is fixed to the floor while instruments give the impression of flight) became quite sophisticated during the jet age, allowing new pilots to not only learn and practice normal instrument procedures, but also to handle a wide variety of airborne emergencies. By the age of jumbo jets, supersonic airliners, and space shuttles, "full motion" simulators gave the illusion of true flight and pilots could actually look out the window and "take off" and "land" at any airport in the world. And the U.S. military now uses sophisticated training simulators, with 10-channel sound effects, voice recognition software (including the languages of potential enemies and allies), and battle smells (via burnt charcoal) to prepare troops for war.

These kinds of training and performance evaluation aids—where the trainees interact with other human beings as well as with machinery and virtual displays—may hold the highest potential for medical simulations, which to date have been pretty primitive. For decades, doctors practiced giving injections to oranges and learned suturing on pig's feet. A somewhat lifelike mannequin (nicknamed "Annie," for unknown reasons) has been used for years to teach cardiopulmonary resuscitation (CPR). Recently, these training mannequins have become more realistic, allowing students to deliver electric shocks with defibrillator paddles and note changes to heart rhythms, insert intravenous and intra-arterial lines, and perform intubations (Figure 17–1). Surgical simulators are beginning to be used both to provide basic practice for medical students and residents and to help experienced surgeons learn new techniques. The major hurdle for these systems is simulating the feel of real flesh, but even that obstacle is being overcome with new technologies and materials.

For most medical operations, the link between improved dexterity from simulator training and fewer errors remains intuitively attractive but not yet fully proven.[8,9] In the absence of hard proof, and because they are

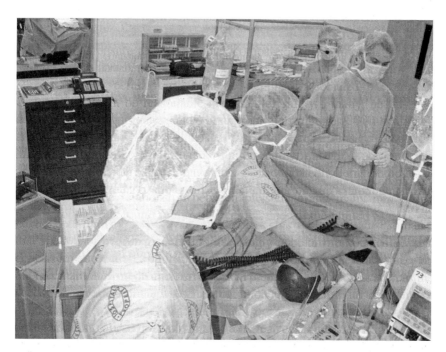

FIGURE 17–1.   A modern high fidelity simulator. (Reproduced with permission from http://anesthesia.stanford.edu/ VASimulator/.)

expensive (some surgical simulators run over 100,000 dollars), the broad dissemination of simulator training will depend on regulatory requirements, cost-sharing (e.g., some regions and professional societies have formed consortia to purchase simulators), and return-on-investment considerations. One study showed that because novice surgeons are slower in the operating room (OR) and require substantial hand-holding by senior physicians, an average of 50,000 dollars in precious OR time is "wasted" during each resident's 4-year training period.[10] In the end, the arguments for using simulators prior to the "real thing" may hinge as much on clinical efficiency as safety.

Although one study showed that trainees improved as much on a urologic simulator that cost less than a dollar (rubber tubes standing in for the urethra, styrofoam cup for the bladder) as a high-tech version costing tens of thousands of dollars,[11] the direction is clearly toward more realistic, technologically sophisticated simulators. Modern virtual reality simulators are beginning to input actual human data, such as that drawn from an extraordinarily detailed digitized cadaver model known as the "Visible Human." Other simulators are being developed that, rather than using generic anatomical data such as from the Visible Human, use real patients' anatomy from computed tomography (CT) or magnetic resonance imaging (MRI) scans. The day may come when surgeons will walk-through their patient's operation (based on actual anatomy) before a complex surgery.

While it is easy to get excited about this futuristic technology, simulators are unlikely to ever completely replace having a well-prepared young learner observing, then doing, then being corrected by a seasoned veteran. The line between learning and doing will be further blurred as simulations become more realistic and real surgeries become less invasive and more like the simulations. As more and more surgeries and procedures become "virtual," it will be important to remember that simulators can help augment trainees' technical competence, but are highly unlikely to fully replace the need for trainees to learn their craft—as safely as possible—with real patients.

KEY POINTS

- Medical training has always had to balance autonomy and oversight, and has traditionally tipped this balance toward trainee autonomy, partly for economic reasons.

- Driven in large part by the patient safety movement, this balance is tipping back toward oversight, reflected in more available and involved supervisors and efforts to encourage trainees to admit their limitations and call for help.

- Particularly in procedural fields, the use of simulation will help trainees traverse their learning curves with fewer risks to patients.

REFERENCES

1. Gawande AA. *Complications: A Surgeon's Notes on an Imperfect Science.* New York, NY: Henry Holt and Company, 2002.
2. Robins N. *The Girl who Died Twice: Every Patient's Nightmare: The Libby Zion Case and the Hidden Hazards of Hospitals.* New York, NY: Delacorte Press, 1995.
3. Wu AW, Folkman S, McPhee SJ, et al. Do house officers learn from their mistakes? *JAMA* 1991;265:2089–2094.
4. Shojania KG, Fletcher KE, Saint S. Graduate medical education and patient safety: a busy—and occasionally hazardous—intersection. *Ann Intern Med* 2006;145:592–598.
5. Wachter RM, Shojania KG. *Internal Bleeding: The Truth Behind America's Terrifying Epidemic of Medical Mistakes.* New York, NY: Rugged Land, 2004.
6. Moore MJ, Bennett CL. The learning curve for laparoscopic cholecystectomy. The Southern Surgeons Club. *Am J Surg* 1995;170:55–59.
7. Morino M, Festa V, Garrone C. Survey on Torino courses. The impact of a two-day practical course on apprenticeship and diffusion of laparoscopic cholecystectomy in Italy. *Surg Endosc* 1995;9:46–48.
8. Salas E, Wilson KA, Burke CS, et al. Using simulation-based training to improve patient safety: what does it take? *Jt Comm J Qual Patient Saf* 2005;31:363–371.
9. Sutherland LM, Middleton PF, Anthony A. Surgical simulation: a systematic review. *Ann Surg* 2006;243:291–300.
10. Bridges M, Diamond DL. The financial impact of teaching surgical residents in the operating room. *Am J Surg* 1999;177:28–32.
11. Matsumoto ED, Hamstra SJ, Radomski SB, et al. The effect of bench model fidelity on endourological skills: a randomized controlled study. *J Urol* 2002; 167:2354–2357.

ADDITIONAL READINGS

Amalberti R, Auroy Y, Berwick D, et al. Five system barriers to achieving ultrasafe health care. *Ann Intern Med* 2005;142:756–764.
Bosk CL. *Forgive and Remember: Managing Medical Failure*, 2nd ed. Chicago, IL: University of Chicago Press, 2003.

Christensen JF, Levinson W, Dunn PM. The heart of darkness: the impact of perceived mistakes on physicians. *J Gen Intern Med* 1992;7:424–431.

Moorthy K, Munz Y, Forrest D, et al. Surgical crisis management skills training and assessment: a simulation-based approach to enhancing operating room performance. *Ann Surg* 2006;244:139–147.

Wachter RM. Expected and unanticipated consequences of the quality and information technology revolutions. *JAMA* 2006;295:2780–2783.

CHAPTER EIGHTEEN

The Malpractice System

OVERVIEW

A *middle-aged woman was admitted to the medical ward with a moderate case of pneumonia. After being started promptly on antibiotics and fluids, she clinically stabilized for a few hours. But she deteriorated overnight, leading to symptoms and signs of severe hypoxemia and septic shock. The nurse paged a young physician, working the overnight shift, to see the patient. The doctor arrived within minutes. She found the patient confused, hypotensive, tachypnic, and hypoxic. Oxygen brought the patient's oxygen saturation up to the low 90s, and the doctor now had a difficult choice to make. The patient, confused and agitated, clearly had respiratory failure: the need for intubation and mechanical ventilation was obvious. But should the young doctor intubate the patient on the floor or quickly transport her to the ICU, a few floors below, where the experienced staff could perform the intubation more safely? Part of this trade-off was the doctor's awareness of her own limitations. She had performed only a handful of intubations in her career, most under the guidance of an anesthesiologist in an unhurried setting, and the ward nurses also lacked experience in helping with the procedure. A third option was to call an ICU team to the ward, but that could take as long as transferring the patient downstairs.*

After thinking about it for a moment, she made her choice: bring the patient promptly to the ICU. She called the Unit to be ready. "In my mind it was a matter of what would be safest," she reflected later. And so the doctor, a floor nurse, and a respiratory

199

therapist wheeled the patient's bed to the elevator, and then to the ICU. Unfortunately, in the ten minutes between notifying the ICU and arriving there the patient's condition markedly worsened, and she was in extremis when she arrived. After an unsuccessful urgent intubation attempt, the patient became pulseless. Frantically now, one doctor shocked the patient while another prepared to reattempt intubation. On the third shock, the patient's heart restarted and the intubation was completed. The patient survived, but was left with severe hypoxic brain damage.

The young physician apologized to the family, more out of empathy than guilt. In her mind, she had made the right decisions at the right time, despite the terrible outcome.

Nearly two years later, the physician received notice that she was being sued by the patient's family, alleging negligence in delaying the intubation. The moment she received the news is seared in her memory—just like those terrible moments spent trying to save the patient whose family was now seeking to punish her. "I was sitting in the ICU" she said, "and my partner calls me up and says, 'You're being sued . . . and that's why I'm leaving medicine'."[1]

TORT LAW AND THE MALPRACTICE SYSTEM

The need to compensate people for their injuries has long been recognized in most systems of law, and Western systems have traditionally done so by apportioning fault (*culpa*). *Tort law*, the general legal discipline that includes malpractice law (as well as product liability and personal injury law) takes these two principles—compensating the injured in an effort to "make them whole" and making the party "at fault" responsible for this restitution—and weaves them into a single system. The linking of compensation of the injured to the fault of the injurer is brilliant in its simplicity and works reasonably well when applied to many human endeavors.[2]

Unfortunately, medicine is not one of them. Because most errors involve slips—glitches in automatic behaviors that can strike even the most conscientious practitioner (Chapter 2)—they are unintentional and cannot be deterred by threat of lawsuits. Moreover, as the rest of the book has hopefully made clear, in most circumstances the doctor or nurse holding the smoking gun is not truly "at fault," but simply the last in line in a long error chain.

This discussion is not referring to the acts of providers who fail to adhere to expected standards and whose slips, therefore, are not unintentional errors, but predictable damage wrought by unqualified, unmotivated, or reckless workers. These situations will be discussed more fully in the next chapter, but the malpractice system (coupled with more vigorous efforts to hold the providers accountable and protect future patients) seems appropriate in dealing with such caregivers. An analogy might be the difference between a driver who accidentally hits a child who darts into traffic chasing a ball, and a drunk driver who hits a child on the sidewalk after losing control of his speeding car. Both accidents result in death, but the second driver is clearly more culpable. If the malpractice system confined its wrath to medicine's version of the drunk, speeding driver—particularly the repeat offender—it would be difficult to criticize it. But that is not the case.

Consider a doctor who performs a risky and difficult surgical procedure, and has done it safely thousands of time but finally slips. The injured patient sues, claiming that the doctor didn't adhere to the "standard of care." A defense argument that the surgeon normally *did* avoid the error, or that some errors are a statistical inevitability if you do a complex procedure often enough, holds little water in the malpractice system, which makes it fundamentally unfair to those whose jobs cause them to frequently engage in risky activities. As Alan Merry, a New Zealand anesthesiologist, and Alexander McCall Smith, an accomplished novelist and Professor of Medical Law at the University of Edinburgh, observe, "All too often the yardstick is taken to be the person who is capable of meeting a high standard of competence, awareness, care, etc., *all the time.* Such a person is unlikely to be human."[2]

The same is true of judgment calls, such as the one the physician made in choosing to take her septic patient to the ICU. Such difficult calls come up all the time. Because the tort system reviews them only after the fact, it creates a powerful instinct to assign blame (of course, we can never know what would have happened had the physician chosen to intubate the patient on the ward). "The tendency in such circumstances is to praise a decision if it proves successful and to call it 'an error of judgment' if not," write Merry and Smith. "Success is its own justification; failure needs a great deal of explanation."

How can judges and juries (and patients and providers) avoid the distorting effects of hindsight and deal more fairly with caregivers doing their best under difficult conditions? Safety expert James Reason recommends the *Johnston Substitution Test*, which does not compare an act to an arbitrary standard of excellence, but asks only if a similarly qualified caregiver in the same situation would have behaved any differently. If the answer is, "probably not," then, as the test's inventor Neil Johnston puts it, "Apportioning blame has no material role to play, other than to obscure systemic deficiencies and to blame one of the victims."[3,4]

Liability seems more justified when rules or principles have been violated, since these usually do involve conscious choices by caregivers. But—in healthcare at least—even rule violations may not automatically merit blame. For example, even generally rule-abiding physicians and nurses will periodically need to violate certain rules (e.g., proscriptions against verbal orders are often violated when compliance would cause unnecessary patient suffering, such as when a patient urgently requires analgesia). That is not to condone healthcare anarchy—routine rule violations should cause us to rethink the rule in question, and some rules (like "sign your site"; Chapter 5) should never be broken. But the malpractice system will seize upon evidence that a rule was broken when there is a bad outcome, ignoring the fact that some particular rules are broken by nearly everyone in the name of efficiency—or sometimes even quality and safety (Chapter 4).

Tort law is fluid: Every society must decide how to set the bar regarding fault and compensation. By mating the recompense of the injured to the finding of fault, tort systems inevitably lower the fault-finding bar to allow for easier compensation of sympathetic victims. But this is not the only reason the bar tilts toward fault finding. Humans (particularly of the American variety) tend to be unsettled by vague "systems" explanations, and even more unsettled by the possibility that a horrible outcome could have been "no one's fault." Moreover, the continuing erosion of professional privilege and a questioning of all things "expert" (driven by the media, the Internet, and more) has further tipped the balance between plaintiff and defendant. But it was already an unfair match: Faced with the heart-wrenching story of an injured patient or grieving family, who can possibly swallow an explanation that "things like this just happen" and that no one is to blame, especially when the potential source of compensation is a "rich doctor," or an insurance company?[5]

The role of the expert witness further tips the already lopsided scales of malpractice justice. Almost by definition, expert witnesses (truth in advertising: I have been an expert witness on approximately 20 cases, for both plaintiffs and defendants) are particularly well informed about their areas of expertise, which makes it exceptionally difficult for them to assume the mindset of "the reasonable practitioner," especially as the case becomes confrontational and experts gravitate to more polarized positions.

Finally, adding to the confusion is the fact that doctors and nurses feel guilty for our errors (even when there was no true fault), often blaming ourselves because we failed to live up to our own expectation of perfection. Just as naturally, what person would not instinctively lash out against a provider when faced with a brain-damaged child or spouse. It is to be expected that families or patients will blame the party holding the smoking gun, just as they would a driver who struck their child who ran into the street to get a ball. Some bereaved families (and drivers and doctors) will ultimately move on to a deeper understanding that no one is to blame—that the tragedy is just that. But whether they do or do not, write Merry and Smith, "It is essential that the law should do so."[2]

If the malpractice system unfairly assigns fault when there is none, what really is the harm, other than the payment of a few (or a few million) dollars by physicians, hospitals, or insurance companies to injured patients and families? I believe that there *is* harm, particularly as we try to engage rank-and-file physicians in patient safety efforts. Physicians, particularly in high-risk malpractice fields (such as obstetrics and neurosurgery) are increasingly demoralized and depressed, and providers in this sour mood are unlikely to be enthusiastic patient safety leaders. Tort law is adversarial by nature, while a culture of safety is collaborative (Chapter 15). In a safety-conscious culture, doctors and nurses willingly report their mistakes as opportunities to make themselves and the system better (Chapter 14), something they are unlikely to do in a litigious environment.

This is not to say—as some do—that the malpractice system has done nothing to improve patient safety. Defensive medicine is not necessarily a bad thing, and some of the defensive measures taken by doctors and hospitals make sense. Anesthesiologists now continuously monitor patients' oxygen levels, which has been partly responsible for vastly improved surgical safety (and remarkable decreases in anesthesiologists' malpractice premiums) (Chapter 5). Nurses and physicians keep better records than they would without the malpractice system. Informed consent, driven partly by malpractice considerations, can give patients the opportunity to think twice about procedures and have their questions answered (Chapter 21).

Unfortunately, in other ways, "defensive medicine" is a shameful waste, particularly when there are so many unmet healthcare needs. A 1996 study estimated that limiting pain and suffering awards would trim healthcare costs by 5–9% by reducing unnecessary and expensive tests, diminishing referrals to unneeded specialists, and so on.[6] In today's dollars, these saving would amount to over 250 billion dollars yearly in the United States.

In the last analysis, though, it is the way in which our legal system misrepresents medical errors that is its most damning legacy. By focusing attention on smoking guns and individual providers, a lawsuit creates the illusion of making care safer without actually doing so. Doctors in Canada are five times less likely to be sued than American doctors, for example, but there is no evidence that they commit fewer errors.[1,7] And a 1990 study by Brennan demonstrated an almost total disconnect between the malpractice process and efforts to improve quality in hospitals. Of 82 cases handled by risk managers (as a result of the possibility of a lawsuit) in which quality problems were involved, only 12 (15%) were even discussed by the doctors at their departmental quality meetings or Morbidity and Mortality (M&M) conferences.[8]

What people often find most shocking about America's malpractice system is that it does not even serve the needs of injured patients. Despite stratospheric malpractice premiums, generous settlements, big awards by sympathetic juries, and an epidemic of defensive medicine, many patients with "compensable injuries" remain uncompensated. In fact, less than 3% of patients who experience injuries associated with negligent care file claims. The reasons for this are varied, and include patients' unawareness that an error occurred, the fact that most cases are taken by attorneys on contingency (and thus will not be brought if the attorneys feel that their investment in preparing the case is unlikely to be recouped), and the fact that many of the un- or undercompensated claimants are on government assistance and lack the resources, personal initiative, or social clout to seek redress. Thus, some worthy malpractice claims go begging while others go forward for a host of reasons that have nothing to do with the presence or degree of negligence.

Finally, even when injured patients' cases do make it through the malpractice system to a trial or settlement, it is remarkable how little money actually ends up in the hands of the victims and their families. After deducting legal fees and expenses, the average plaintiff sees about 40 cents for every dollar paid by the defendant. If the intent of the award is to help families care for a permanently disabled relative or to replace a deceased breadwinner's earnings, this 60% overhead makes the malpractice system a uniquely wasteful business.

NO-FAULT SYSTEMS: AN ALTERNATIVE TO TORT-BASED MALPRACTICE

Studies by Brennan and colleagues have shown that doctors have a more than 1-in-100 chance of being tagged with a lawsuit after a patient has an adverse event, even when the doctor has done nothing wrong.[9,10] Although this may not sound like an excessive "risk" of a lawsuit, when you consider all the patients who suffer adverse events (e.g., medication side effects, complications after surgery), this rate adds up to a lot of suits. Over a career, the average doctor can nearly count on being sued at least once, and far more than that in the riskier specialties.

What types of cases trigger the most malpractice suits and yield the biggest awards? In Brennan's studies, the magnitude of the patient's disability was by far a better predictor of victory and award size than was proof of a breach of "standard of care." In other words, the American malpractice system distributes compensation according to the degree of injury, not the degree of malpractice.

This is not altogether surprising, because malpractice cases are generally heard by juries composed of ordinary citizens who tend to be sympathetic to people like them who have been harmed. The defendant's talk about standards of care and probabilistic outcomes are a tough sell when stacked up against a dead or horribly disabled plaintiff. "In a case like this," said the attorney who represented the physician in the case that began this chapter, "involving a patient who was already in the hospital, who has an arrest and anoxic [brain damage], one of the very significant perceptual issues we have to consider... is the fact that there was a catastrophic outcome, and to some jurors, catastrophic outcomes may equate with 'somebody must have messed up'."[1] And so, despite expert testimony that the doctor's decision to postpone intubation was medically sound, the attorney advised his client to settle out of court, which she did. The frequency of this outcome—even when the physician feels she was anything but negligent—provides an incentive for more lawsuits.

Given the problems in the American malpractice system, pain-and-suffering caps (first implemented in the State of California after a malpractice crisis in the 1980s) have been touted as a way of at least moderating insurance premiums and keeping doctors in business.[11] However, they don't solve the fundamental problem. Physicians worry more about the costs—both financial and psychic—of the process than the costs of the settlement. If a patient comes to us with a headache and, after a conscientious workup, we conclude it is almost certainly not a brain tumor, we reassure the patient and look for other diagnoses. However, if 1 out of every 5000 times a patient *does* have a brain tumor and we skipped the computed axial tomography (CAT) scan, we can count on being sued. In that case, the expense and emotional costs—time lost to depositions, hand-wringing and demoralization, sleepless nights, and suppressed anger over the inherent unfairness of it all—is essentially the same for the physician whether the payout is 400,000 or 2 million dollars. As doctors, our decision-making is driven more by the potential for being sued than by the cost of losing a judgment.

Brennan, Studdert, and colleagues have made a strong case for replacing the adversarial tort-based malpractice approach with a no-fault system modeled on workers' compensation.[1,12] A no-fault pool would be created from insurance premiums from which awards would be made following the simple establishment of harm to the patient at the hands of the medical system. There would be no need to prove that the caregiver was negligent or the care was substandard. The proposed advantages of the system include more rapid adjudication of cases, and far lower overhead (to lawyers, expert witnesses, and so on).

There are many concerns about the viability and political feasibility of a no-fault system in the United States, and setting the bar for compensation will be challenging (too low, such as compensation for a gastrointestinal bleed after appropriate use of a nonsteroidal anti-inflammatory agent, and the system will rapidly go broke; too high (e.g., payouts restricted to horrible "Never Events"; Appendix VI) and too many people suffering significant harm will go uncompensated). Although some worry about the loss of a deterrent effect, the evidence supporting such an effect in our current malpractice system is quite limited.[1] And, in Brennan's scheme, institutions would be "experience rated" (i.e., their premiums would be set based on their payout histories), providing an incentive to create and maintain safe systems of care.

The debate continues in the United States, driven more by political than policy considerations. The experience from other countries provides a mixed but generally favorable record. New Zealand, for example, switched to a no-fault system for *all* personal injuries, including healthcare-related, in 1972. The no-fault system is seen as a partial success, although there has been agitation for a more fault-based system to deal with egregious errors.[2,13] The Swedish no-fault system remains effective and popular after more than two decades. Sweden limits compensable events to medical injuries that were "avoidable"; and eligible patients must have spent at least 10 days in the hospital or endured at least 30 sick days.[2,12,14]

So for now, the American malpractice system remains highly unpopular, with few judging that it fairly assesses blame or compensates victims.[15] From the standpoint of patient safety, its main problems are that it creates an adversarial environment that encourages secrecy rather than the openness necessary for problem solving, and that it tends to point fingers at people rather than focus on systems defects. But there seems little hope that the system will give way to a better one anytime in the foreseeable future.

KEY POINTS

- The medical malpractice system in the United States is governed by the rules of tort law, which compensates victims of injuries with the resources of at-fault providers.

- Among the criticisms of the malpractice system are its arbitrariness, its high administrative costs, and its tendency to assign individual blame rather than seek systems solutions. The latter issue in particular often places the malpractice system in conflict with the goals of the patient safety movement.

- Pain and suffering award caps can help limit the size of awards and decrease the propensity of attorneys to accept cases on contingency, but do not improve the fundamental flaws in the system.

- Recently, no-fault systems, in which patients are compensated based on injuries without the need to assign fault, have been promoted in the United States. Early international experiences with such systems have been generally positive.

REFERENCES

1. Brennan TA, Mello MM. Patient safety and medical malpractice: a case study. *Ann Intern Med* 2003;139:267–273.
2. Merry A, McCall Smith A. *Errors, Medicine, and the Law.* Cambridge, England: Cambridge University Press, 2001.
3. Johnston N. Do blame and punishment have a role in organizational risk management? *Flight Deck* 1995;Spring:33–36.
4. Reason JT. *Managing the Risks of Organizational Accidents.* Aldershot, Hampshire, England: Ashgate, 1997.
5. Wachter RM, Shojania KG. *Internal Bleeding: The Truth Behind America's Terrifying Epidemic of Medical Mistakes.* New York, NY: Rugged Land, 2004.
6. Kessler DP, McClellan M. Do doctors practice defensive medicine? *Q J Econ* 1996;111:353–390.
7. Blendon RJ, Schoen C, DesRoches CM, et al. Confronting competing demands to improve quality: a five-country hospital survey. *Health Aff (Millwood)* 2004;23:119–135.

8. Brennan TA, Localio AR, Leape LL, et al. Identification of adverse events occurring during hospitalization. A cross-sectional study of litigation, quality assurance, and medical records at two teaching hospitals. *Ann Intern Med* 1990;112:221–226.

9. Localio AR, Lawthers AG, Brennan TA, et al. Relation between malpractice claims and adverse events due to negligence. Results of the Harvard Medical Practice Study III. *N Engl J Med* 1991;325:245–251.

10. Studdert DM, Thomas EJ, Burstin HR, et al. Negligent care and malpractice claiming behavior in Utah and Colorado. *Med Care* 2000;38:250–260.

11. Hellinger FJ, Encinosa WE. The impact of state laws limiting malpractice damage awards on health care expenditures. *Am J Public Health* 2006; 96:1375–1381.

12. Studdert DM, Brennan TA. No-fault compensation for medical injuries: the prospect for error prevention. *JAMA* 2001;286:217–223.

13. Bismark MM, Brennan TA, Patterson RJ, et al. Relationship between complaints and quality of care in New Zealand: a descriptive analysis of complainants and non-complainants following adverse events. *Qual Saf Health Care* 2006;15:17–22.

14. Mello MM, Studdert DM, Kachalia AB, et al. "Health courts" and accountability for patient safety. *Milbank Q* 2006;84:459–492.

15. Gawande AA. The malpractice mess. *New Yorker* 2005:62–71.

ADDITIONAL READINGS

Gawande A. *Complications: A Surgeon's Notes on an Imperfect Science*. New York, NY: Metropolitan Books, 2002.

Kachalia A, Shojania KG, Hofer TP, et al. Does full disclosure of medical errors affect malpractice liability? The jury is still out. *Jt Comm J Qual Saf* 2003;29:503–511.

Studdert DM, Mello MM, Gawande AA, et al. Disclosure of medical injury to patients: an improbable risk management strategy. *Health Aff (Millwood)* 2007;26:215–226.

Studdert DM, Mello MM, Gawande AA, et al. Claims, errors, and compensation payments in medical malpractice litigation. *N Engl J Med* 2006; 354:2024–2033.

Wachter RM. The end of the beginning: patient safety five years after "To Err is Human." *Health Aff (Millwood)* 2004;(Suppl W4):534–545.

CHAPTER NINETEEN

Accountability

OVERVIEW

As the entire book has made clear, the fundamental underpinning of the modern patient safety field is "systems thinking"—the notion that most errors are made by competent, caring people, and that patient safety therefore depends on embedding providers in systems that anticipate errors and block them from causing harm. That is an attractive viewpoint, and undoubtedly correct in the main. But it risks averting our eyes from those providers or institutions who, for a variety of reasons, are not competent, or worse. This chapter will discuss the issue of accountability, reflecting a bit on its most visible incarnation, the malpractice system (Chapter 18), and other ways that accountability can be exercised. We will return in the end to the fundamental question: can the desire for "no blame" be reconciled with the need for accountability?

ACCOUNTABILITY

Scott Torrence (all names are pseudonyms), a 36-year-old insurance broker, was struck in the head while going up for a rebound during his weekend basketball game. Over the next few hours, a mild headache escalated into a thunderclap, and he became lethargic and vertiginous. His girlfriend called an ambulance to take him to the emergency room in his local rural hospital, which lacked a CAT or MRI scanner. The ER physician, Dr. Jane Benamy, worried about brain bleeding, called neurologist Dr. Roy Jones at the regional referral hospital (a few hundred miles away) requesting that Torrence be transferred. Jones refused, reassuring Benamy that the case sounded like "benign positional vertigo." Benamy worried, but had no recourse. She sent Torrence home with medications for vertigo and headache.

The next morning, Benamy reevaluated Torrence, and he was markedly worse, with more headache pain, more vertigo, and now vomiting and photophobia (bright lights hurt his eyes). She called neurologist Jones again, who again refused the request for transfer. Completely frustrated, she hospitalized Torrence for intravenous pain medications and close observation.

The next day, the patient was even worse. Literally begging, Benamy found another physician (an internist named Soloway) at Regional Medical Center to accept the transfer, and Torrence was sent there by air ambulance. The CAT scan at Regional was read as unrevealing (in retrospect, a subtle but crucial abnormality was overlooked), and Soloway managed Torrence's symptoms with more pain medicines and sedation. Overnight, however, the patient deteriorated even further—"awake, moaning, yelling," according to the nursing notes—and needed to be physically restrained. Soloway called the neurologist, Dr. Jones, at home, who told him that he "was familiar with the case and . . . the non-focal neurological exam and the normal CAT scan made urgent clinical problems unlikely." He went on to say that "he would evaluate the patient the next morning."

But by the next morning, Torrence was dead. An autopsy revealed that the head trauma had torn a small cerebellar artery, which led to a cerebellar stroke (an area of the brain poorly imaged by CAT scan). Ultimately, the stroke caused enough swelling to trigger brainstem herniation—extrusion of the brain through one of the holes in the base of the skull, like toothpaste squeezing through a tube. This cascade of falling dominoes could have been stopped at any stage, but that would have required the expert neurologist to see the patient, recognize the signs of the cerebellar artery dissection, take a closer look at the CAT scan, and order an MRI.[1]

Cases like this one—specifically Dr. Jones's refusal to personally evaluate a challenging and rapidly deteriorating patient when asked by concerned colleagues to do so on multiple occasions—demonstrate the tension between the "no fault" stance embraced by the patient safety field and the importance of establishing and enforcing standards. That such cases occur should not surprise anyone. Despite years of training, doctors are as vulnerable as anyone to all the maladies that can beset professionals in high-demand, rapidly changing professions: not keeping up, drug and alcohol abuse, depression, burnout, or just failing to care enough.

But how can we reconcile the need for accountability with our desire to shift from "blame and shame" to a new focus on system safety? As Dr. Lucian Leape, the Harvard surgeon and father of the modern patient safety movement, lamented:

> There is no accountability. When we identify doctors who harm patients, we need to try to be compassionate and help them. But in the end, if they are a danger to patients, they shouldn't be caring for them. A fundamental principle has to be the development and then the enforcement of procedures and standards. We can't make real progress without them. When a doctor doesn't follow them, something has to happen. Today, nothing does, and you have a vicious cycle in which people have no real incentive to follow the rules because they know there are no consequences if they don't. So there *are* bad doctors and bad nurses, but the fact that we tolerate them is just another systems problem.[1]

One of the definitions of a profession is that it sets its own standards and is therefore self-policing. Yet it is undeniable that doctors and hospitals do have a tendency to protect their own, sometimes at the expense of patients. Hospital "credentials committees," which certify and periodically recertify individual doctors, rarely limit a provider's privileges, even when there is stark evidence of failure to meet a reasonable standard of care. If alcohol or drug abuse is the problem, the physician may be ordered to enter a "diversion" program, a noble idea, but one that sometimes errs on the side of protecting the interests of the dangerous provider over an unwitting public.

Why has healthcare failed to live up to its ethical mandate to self-regulate? One reason is that it is difficult to sanction one's own peers, especially when the evidence of substandard practice is anecdotal and sometimes concerns issues of personality (i.e., the disruptive physician, or the physician who appears to be insufficiently responsive) rather than "hard outcomes." A second issue is more practical: given the length of time that it takes to train physicians, committees and licensing bodies are understandably reluctant to remove a physician's privileges after they and the community have invested so much money and effort in training them. A final reason is that physicians tend not to be strong organizational managers. Unlike fields like law and business, in which conflict and competition are commonplace, physicians are generally not used to confronting colleagues, let alone managing the regulatory and legal consequences of such confrontations. This final point is important: because litigation often follows any challenges to a physician's clinical competence (and credentials committee members are only partially shielded from lawsuits), many physicians understandably will do backflips to avoid confrontation.

Unfortunately, the evidence that there *are* bad apples—and that they are not dealt with effectively—is relatively strong. For example, from 1990 to 2002, just 5% of U.S. doctors were involved in 54% of the payouts reported to the National Practitioner Data Bank, the confidential log of malpractice cases maintained by the federal government. Of the 35,000 doctors with two or more payouts, only 8% were disciplined by state boards. And among the 2774 doctors who had made payments in five or more cases, only 463 (just one out of six) had been disciplined. One Pennsylvania doctor paid a whopping 24 claims totaling 8 million dollars between 1993 and 2001, including a wrong-site surgery and a retained instrument case, yet had not been stripped of his clinical credentials nor disciplined by the state licensing board.[2]

Of course, in this group of oft-sued doctors are some very busy obstetricians and neurosurgeons who take on tough cases (probably accompanied by poor bedside manner—there is a striking correlation between the number of patient complaints about a physician's personal style and the probability of lawsuits[3]). But this group undoubtedly also includes some very dangerous doctors. It will be important to find better ways to measure whether doctors are meeting those standards (the increasing computerization of practice will help by making it much easier to tell whether docs are practicing high-quality, evidence-based medicine). Moreover, efforts at remediation (and discipline, if necessary) must begin early: one study found that evidence of unprofessional behavior in medical school was a powerful predictor of subsequent disciplinary action by medical boards, often decades later.[4]

While the above discussion has emphasized the quality of physician care, similar issues arise with other health professionals. In these other fields, however, there has been a tradition of more accountability, in part because nurses often work for institutions such as hospitals (and therefore can be more easily fired) and because they have less power. Nevertheless, here too there are problems. The bar for competence and performance should be set similarly high for all healthcare professionals, and the consequences of failing to meet standards should also be similar.[5] Nothing undermines an institution's claim to be committed to safety more than for frontline workers to see that there is one set of standards for nurses, and a wholly different one for physicians.

In this regard, a major change over the past few years has been the development of critical safety rules and standards. Whereas concerns about professional performance in the past largely centered on clinical competence (i.e., frequent diagnostic errors, poor surgical skill), they increasingly relate to failure to adhere to standards and regulations. For example, what should be done about the physician who chooses not to perform a "time out" prior to surgery (Chapter 5)? Or the nurse who habitually fails to clean her hands before patient contact (Chapter 10)? In the end, healthcare organizations must find the strength to enforce these rules and standards, recognizing that there is no conflict between this tough love stance and the "systems approach" to patient safety because some errors—particularly willful and repeated violations of sensible safety rules—are indeed blameworthy. As safety expert James Reason says of habitual rule benders:

> Seeing them get away with it on a daily basis does little for morale or for the credibility of the disciplinary system. Watching them getting their "come-uppance" is not only satisfying, it also serves to reinforce where the boundaries of acceptable behavior lie . . . Justice works two ways. Severe sanctions for the few can protect the innocence of the many.[6]

Moreover, there are cases of such egregious deviations from professional norms that the perpetrators *must* be held accountable in the name of justice and patient protection. Take the case of the Saskatchewan anesthetist convicted of criminal negligence for leaving the operating room to make a phone call (after disconnecting the ventilator alarms), leading to permanent brain injury in a 17-year-old patient,[7] or the Boston surgeon who left his patient anesthetized on the table with a gaping incision in his back to go cash a check at his local bank.[8] And even these cases pale in comparison to those of psychopathic serial killers like Dr. Michael Swango and Dr. Harold Shipman.[9,10] These cases literally beg for justice and accountability, but they are by far the exception, which is what makes the issue of exercising appropriate accountability so vexing.

THE ROLE OF THE MEDIA

Many people look to the media to shine a light on the problem of patient safety and to ensure accountability. The thinking goes that such transparency (sometimes driven by mandated public reporting of errors; see

Chapters 3 and 14) will create a powerful business case for safety, drive hospitals and providers toward enforcing rules and standards, and generate the resources needed to catalyze needed systems change. And there is no doubt that such scrutiny can have precisely this effect—it is difficult to find hospitals or health systems as energized as those with the misfortune to have had highly public errors (Table 1–1).

But while the patient safety efforts at institutions like Johns Hopkins, Duke, and Dana-Farber were clearly turbocharged by mediagenic errors, media scrutiny can also tap into institutional and individual fear of public disclosure and spur an atmosphere of silence. Such a response increases the chance that providers and organizations will fail to discuss and learn from their own errors. Although this response is largely a product of the culture and leadership of each organization (Chapters 15 and 22), the way the media chooses to handle errors can influence the way healthcare organizations respond to the prospect of media attention. The more distorted the coverage (e.g., emphasizing bad apples over systems), the more harmful the effect is likely to be. Over the past few years, many media reports of medical errors have reflected a much more sophisticated understanding of the issues, which increases the probability that the reports will help more than harm.[11]

RECONCILING "NO BLAME" AND ACCOUNTABILITY

The balancing act is a tricky one—in our zeal to replace the malpractice system with another, more rational forum for accountability, we need to guard against creating overly punitive and aggressive licensing boards and credentials committees. After all, the fundamental underpinning of patient safety remains caregiver trust that raising concerns about dysfunctional systems—through open disclosure of errors and near misses—will catalyze improvements (Chapter 14). An overly punitive system will diminish this kind of open dialogue and exchange, and ultimately harm safety.

So how then to reconcile the tension between "no blame" and "blame." A powerful concept, known as a "*Just Culture,*" has emerged in the last several years. Promoted by an engineer/attorney named David Marx, a Just Culture distinguishes between "human error," "at-risk behavior," and "reckless behavior." Only the latter category, defined as "acting in conscious disregard of substantial and unjustifiable risk," is blameworthy.[12] A number of organizations have found this concept useful as they try to create a culture of accountability while respecting the fundamental need to maintain a system focus and a trusting workforce. The concept is further described in Chapter 15.

KEY POINTS

- Although the systems focus is the (correct) underpinning of the modern patient safety movement, incompetent or dangerous providers and institutions must also be held accountable.
- Healthcare tends to "protect its own," which undermines public trust in the medical professions.
- Vehicles to exercise accountability can be local (such as hospital credentials committees) or outside organizations (such as state licensing boards or national professional organizations).
- The media can play an important role in ensuring accountability, especially if reporting on errors is seen as fair.

REFERENCES

1. Wachter RM, Shojania KG. *Internal Bleeding: The Truth Behind America's Terrifying Epidemic of Medical Mistakes.* New York, NY: Rugged Land, 2004.
2. Wolfe SM. Bad doctors get a free ride. *NY Times (Print)* 2003:A27.
3. Hickson GB, Federspiel CF, Pichert JW, et al. Patient complaints and malpractice risk. *JAMA* 2002;287:2951–2957.
4. Papadakis MA, Teherani A, Banach MA, et al. Disciplinary action by medical boards and prior behavior in medical school. *N Engl J Med* 2005; 353:2673–2682.
5. Johnstone MJ, Kanitsaki O. Processes for disciplining nurses for unprofessional conduct of a serious nature: a critique. *J Adv Nurs* 2005;50:363–371.
6. Reason JT. *Managing the Risks of Organizational Accidents.* Aldershot, Hampshire, England: Ashgate, 1997.
7. Williams LS. Anesthetist receives jail sentence after patient left in vegetative state. *CMAJ* 1995;153:619–620.

8. Anonymous. Surgeon who left an operation to run an errand is suspended. *NY Times (Print)* 2002:A13.

9. Stewart J. *Blind Eye: The Terrifying Story of a Doctor Who Got Away With Murder*. New York, NY: Simon and Schuster, 2000.

10. O'Neill B. Doctor as murderer. Death certification needs tightening up, but it still might not have stopped Shipman. *BMJ* 2000;320:329–330.

11. Millenson ML. Pushing the profession: how the news media turned patient safety into a priority. *Qual Saf Health Care* 2002;11:57–63.

12. Marx D. Patient safety and the "just culture": a primer for health care executives, April 17, 2001. Available at: www.mers-tm.net/support/marx_primer.pdf.

ADDITIONAL READINGS

Dentzer S. Media mistakes in coverage of the Institute of Medicine's error report. *Eff Clin Pract* 2000;3:305–308.

Goldmann D. System failure versus personal accountability—the case for clean hands. *N Engl J Med* 2006;355:121–123.

Lee TH, Meyer GS, Brennan TA. A middle ground on public accountability. *N Engl J Med* 2004;350:2409–2412.

Satava RM. The nature of surgical error: a cautionary tale and a call to reason. *Surg Endosc* 2005;19:1014–1016.

CHAPTER TWENTY

Laws and Regulations

OVERVIEW

W hile one might hope that professionalism and concern for patients would be sufficient incentive to motivate safe behaviors by providers and investments in systems safety by organizations, experience teaches us that they are not. There are simply too many competing pressures for attention and resources, and the nature of safety is that individuals and organizations can often "get away" with bad behavior for long periods of time. Finally, it is unlikely that all providers and institutions will or can keep up with best practices, given a rapidly evolving research base and the never-ending need to keep at least one eye on the bottom line.

These realities create a need for more prescriptive solutions to safety—standards set by external organizations, such as regulatory bodies, payer representatives, and government. This chapter will examine some of these solutions, beginning with regulations and accreditation.

REGULATIONS AND ACCREDITATION

Regulation is "an authoritative rule," while accreditation is a process by which an authoritative body formally recognizes that an organization or a person is competent to carry out specific tasks. Much of what we tend to call regulation is actually accreditation, but takes place in an environment in which a lack of accreditation has nearly the impact of failing to adhere to a regulatory mandate. For example, the *Accreditation Council for Graduate Medical Education* (ACGME), the body that blesses U.S. residency and fellowship programs, is not a regulator but an accreditor.

217

Nevertheless, when the ACGME mandated that residents work less than 80 hours per week in 2003 (Chapter 16), this had the force of regulation, because ACGME has the power to shut programs down for noncompliance.

The most important accreditor in the patient safety field (in the United States) is the *Joint Commission* (previously called the Joint Commission on Accreditation of Healthcare Organizations, or JCAHO). The Joint Commission, which began in 1951 as a joint program of the American College of Surgeons (which began hospital inspections in 1918), the American College of Physicians, the American Hospital Association, the American Medical Association, and the Canadian Medical Association, has become an increasingly powerful force over the last decade by exercising its mandate to improve the safety of American hospitals (and now, through its subsidiary Joint Commission International, hospitals around the world). A list of Joint Commission National Patient Safety Goals, one of the organization's key mechanisms for generating institutional action, is shown in Appendix IV.

In the past, Joint Commission visits to hospitals were announced years in advance. The visits involved a diverse team of trained accreditors (including physicians and nurses) focusing on hospitals' adherence to various policies. Recently, the process has become far more robust: the accreditor's visits now come unannounced, and much of the visit centers around the "Tracer Methodology," a process by which the inspectors follow a given patient's course throughout the hospital, checking documentation of care and speaking to caregivers about their actions and their understanding of safety principles and regulations. In my judgment, this increasingly vigorous approach to safety enforcement has been long in coming, and has markedly improved safety.[1]

Although the Joint Commission does regulate some physicians' offices and ambulatory sites (such as surgery centers), the majority of such sites are either unaccredited or accredited by another organization, such as the American Association for the Accreditation of Ambulatory Surgical Facilities (AAAASF).[2] Over the past few years, concerns have been raised about the safety of ambulatory surgery, in particular, and an increasingly robust set of accreditation standards have been implemented in these environments. But even with this change, the ambulatory environment continues to be far less impacted by the pressures of regulation and accreditation, one of the key differences between patient safety in the inpatient versus office settings (Chapter 12).

Regulation is more potent than accreditation, in that compliance is mandatory (no hospital *has* to be accredited by the Joint Commission, though the vast majority choose to do so) and failure to comply generally carries stiff penalties. Typically, the main regulatory authorities relevant to patient safety are state governments, though there are a few federal regulations and some cities have independent regulations. For example, the State of California now regulates certain nurse-to-patient ratios, and many states now require reporting of certain types of errors to a state entity (Chapters 16 and 14, respectively).

OTHER LEVERS TO PROMOTE SAFETY

Healthcare payers have tremendous power to move the system, though they have not wielded it in the safety arena very aggressively. One exception has been the activities of the *Leapfrog Group*, a healthcare arm of many of America's largest employers (and thus the source of a significant amount of hospital and doctor payments), which was created in part to catalyze patient safety activities. Though Leapfrog has neither accreditation nor regulatory authority, it uses its contracting power to promote safe practices, either through simple transparency or by steering patients toward institutions it deems to be better performers. In 2001, it recommended three "safe practices" (computerized provider order entry [CPOE], favoring high volume providers in areas in which there was evidence linking higher volume to better outcomes [Table 5–1], and having full-time intensivists provide critical care). In 2006, Leapfrog endorsed the National Quality Forum's list of 28 "Never Events" (Appendix VI). There is some evidence that Leapfrog's activities have led to more widespread implementation of the endorsed practices.[3]

Even softer influence has been exercised by professional societies and nonprofit safety-oriented organizations. For example, several professional physician and nursing societies have led campaigns to improve hand hygiene (Chapter 10). In 2005, the *Institute for Healthcare Improvement* (IHI), a nonprofit support and consulting organization, launched a "campaign to save 100,000 lives" by promoting a set of practices in American hospitals[4] (Table 20–1). Although IHI lacks regulatory authority and is not a payer, its campaign succeeded it signing up more than half the hospitals in the United States. This tremendous response was followed in late 2006 by another campaign to "prevent 5 million cases of harm" through another set of safety-oriented practices (Table 20–2). Given the various forces promoting safety in American hospitals, it is difficult to isolate the effect of the IHI campaigns, but there is no doubt that they have captured the attention of the American healthcare system and generated significant change.[5,6]

At the present time, the U.S. healthcare system is embracing transparency (e.g., public reporting of performance) and even experimenting with

TABLE 20–1
The six "planks" in the IHI's 2005–2006 "100,000 Lives Campaign"

Goal	Specific Practices
Prevent ventilator-associated pneumonia	Elevation of the head of the bed Daily "sedation vacation" Peptic ulcer disease prophylaxis Deep venous thrombosis prophylaxis
Prevent central-line-associated bloodstream infections	Hand hygiene Maximal barrier precautions Chlorhexidine skin antisepsis Optimal catheter site selection Daily review of line necessity
Prevent surgical site infections	Appropriate use of antibiotics Appropriate hair removal Perioperative glucose control Perioperative normothermia
Improve care for acute myocardial infarction	Early administration of aspirin Aspirin at discharge Early administration of beta-blocker Beta-blocker at discharge ACE inhibitor or ARB at discharge for patients with systolic dysfunction Timely initiation of reperfusion (thrombolysis or percutaneous coronary intervention) Smoking cessation counseling
Prevent adverse drug events	Medication reconciliation
Deploy Rapid Response Teams	Self-explanatory

Abbreviations: ACE, angiotensin-converting enzyme; ARB, angiotensin-receptor blocker.

differential payments for better performance ("pay for performance").[7–9] The idea behind these efforts is to create a *business case for quality and safety*—a set of incentives generated by patients choosing better and safer providers or providers receiving higher payments for better performance. Although such strategies carry the potential to improve safety as well as quality, it is easier to apply them to quality (process measures such as beta-blockers for patients with myocardial infarction or outcome measures such as risk-adjusted mortality or infection rates) than to safety (medication errors or wrong-site surgery) because of the latter's measurement challenges (Chapter 3).

TABLE 20-2

The six "planks" in the IHI's 2006–2007 campaign to "Protect 5 Million Lives From Harm"

Goal	Specific Practices
Prevent pressure ulcers	Daily inspection of skin from head to toe Keeping the patient dry and treating dry skin with moisturizers Optimizing nutrition and hydration Minimizing pressure through frequent turning and repositioning and through the use of pressure relieving surfaces
Reduce methicillin-resistant *Staphylococcus aureus* (MRSA) infection	Hand hygiene Decontamination of environment and equipment Active surveillance cultures Contact precautions for infected and colonized patients Device bundles (central-line bundle and ventilator bundle)
Prevent harm from high-alert medications (anticoagulants, narcotics and opiates, insulins, and sedatives)	Design processes to prevent errors and harm Design methods to identify errors and harm when they occur Design methods to mitigate the harm that may result from the error
Reduce surgical complications	Surgical site infection prevention Beta-blockers for patients on beta-blockers prior to admission Venous thromboembolism prophylaxis Ventilator-associated pneumonia prevention Improve teamwork and organizational culture
Deliver reliable, evidence-based care for CHF	LVS function assessment ACE inhibitor or ARB at discharge discharge for CHF patients with systolic dysfunction Anticoagulant at discharge for CHF patients with chronic or recurrent atrial fibrillation Smoking cessation advice and counseling Discharge instructions Influenza immunization (seasonal) Pneumococcal immunization
Get boards on board	Governance boards should: Set aims for improvement Get data and hear stories of harm Establish and monitor system-level measures Change the environment, policies, and culture Learning, starting with the board Establish executive accountability

Abbreviations: LVS, left ventricular systolic; CHF, congestive heart failure; ACE, angiotensin-converting enzyme; ARB, angiotensin-receptor blocker.

PROBLEMS WITH REGULATORY AND OTHER PRESCRIPTIVE SOLUTIONS

Since regulators and accreditors have the power to mandate change, why not use these levers more aggressively? Given the toll of medical errors, wouldn't we want to use our biggest, most prescriptive guns?

Perhaps, but regulation, accreditation, and laws are what are known in policy circles as "blunt tools," because of their highly limited abilities to understand local circumstances or institutional culture and calibrate their mandates accordingly. Therefore, they are best used for "low-hanging fruit"—areas amenable to one-size-fits-all solutions, usually because they are not particularly complex and tend not to vary from institution to institution. Examples of such areas might be "sign-your-site" (Chapter 5) and abolition of high-risk abbreviations (Chapter 4): these standards are equally applicable in a 600-bed academic medical center and an 80-bed rural hospital. But as regulation moves into areas that are more nuanced and dependent on cultural changes, the risk of unforeseen consequences increases. For example, medication reconciliation (a patient safety goal introduced by the Joint Commission in 2005), though based on legitimate concerns about medication errors at points of transition (Chapters 4 and 8), has vexed hospitals around the United States because of implementation problems and the absence of published best practices.[10] Leapfrog's mandate that hospitals have CPOE seems reasonable, but it is difficult for the coalition to distinguish between effective and ineffective CPOE (Chapter 13). ACGME's duty hours limits (Chapter 16) have allowed residents to sleep but also created collateral damage by increasing handoffs (Chapter 8). And some nurses have complained that California's mandatory nurse-to-patient ratios have not enhanced safety, because some hospitals have replaced clerical staff or lifting teams to meet the ratios, leaving nurses with no more direct patient care time than they had before the law (Chapter 16).

Despite these limitations, regulation is vital in certain areas, particularly when providers and institutions fail to voluntarily adopt reasonable safety standards. For example, many take-out restaurants have long read back takeout orders to ensure accurate communication (by the way, they did this without a regulatory mandate—their business case to get your takeout order right is powerful enough to motivate the practice), but no healthcare organization mandated this practice until the Joint Commission did so in 2003.[11] Regulation also can standardize practices that should be standardized. For example, prior to the Joint Commission regulations regarding "sign-your-site," many orthopedic surgeons had taken it upon themselves to begin signing limbs in an effort to prevent wrong-site surgery. The problem: some well-meaning surgeons signed the leg *to be operated on* with an X (as in, "cut here"), while others signed the leg *not to be operated on* (as in, "don't cut here"). Obviously, without a standard system for signing the site (the Joint Commission now mandates signing the site *to be operated on*), the opportunity for misunderstanding and errors is great.

Prescriptive tools such as regulations, accreditation standards, and laws have an important role in ensuring patient safety. It is vital that they be used and enforced when they are the right instrument for the job, and that other vehicles (transparency, market forces and competition, social marketing, changes in training, appeals to professionalism, perhaps pay for performance) be used where they are the more appropriate tools.

KEY POINTS

- Regulation and accreditation are powerful tools to promote patient safety in that they can mandate (or nearly mandate) certain practices.

- Other organizations that lack regulatory authority can also catalyze significant change, using levers such as the payment system (as in the case of the Leapfrog Group) or well-established credibility and moral authority (as in the case of the IHI).

- Regulation and accreditation are "blunt tools," and thus are best used for low-hanging fruit: simple processes that are relatively standard independent of organizational size, complexity, and culture. They can be problematic when applied to more complex processes (such as computerization or medication reconciliation).

REFERENCES

1. Wachter RM. The end of the beginning: patient safety five years after "To Err is Human." *Health Aff (Millwood)* 2004; (Suppl W4):534–545.
2. Yates JA. Liposuction gone awry. AHRQ WebM&M (serial online), March 2006. Available at: http://www.webmm.ahrq.gov/case.aspx?caseID=119.
3. Galvin RS, Delbanco S. Why employers need to rethink how they buy health care. *Health Aff (Millwood)* 2005;24:1549–1553.

4. Berwick DM, Calkins DR, McCannon CJ, et al. The 100,000 lives campaign: setting a goal and a deadline for improving health care quality. *JAMA* 2006;295:324–327.
5. Wachter RM, Pronovost PJ. The 100,000 Lives Campaign: a scientific and policy review. *Jt Comm J Qual Patient Saf* 2006;32:621–627, 631–633.
6. Berwick DM, Hackbarth AD, McCannon CJ. IHI replies to "The 100,000 Lives Campaign: a scientific and policy review." *Jt Comm J Qual Patient Saf* 2006;32:628–630; discussion 631–633.
7. Rosenthal MB, Frank RG, Li Z, et al. Early experience with pay-for-performance: from concept to practice. *JAMA* 2005;294:1788–1793.
8. Epstein AM. Paying for performance in the United States and abroad. *N Engl J Med* 2006;355:406–408.
9. Lindenauer PK, Remus D, Roman S, et al. Public reporting and pay for performance in hospital quality improvement. *N Engl J Med* 2007;356: 486–496.
10. Anonymous. Practitioners agree on medication reconciliation value, but frustration and difficulties abound. Institute for Safe Medication Practices Newsletter, July 13, 2006. Available at: http://www.ismp.org/Newsletters/acutecare/articles/20060713.asp.
11. Wachter RM, Shojania KG. *Internal Bleeding: The Truth Behind America's Terrifying Epidemic of Medical Mistakes.* New York, NY: Rugged Land, 2004.

ADDITIONAL READINGS

Brennan TA, Gawande A, Thomas E, et al. Accidental deaths, saved lives, and improved quality. *N Engl J Med* 2005;353:1405–1409.

Devers KJ, Pham HH, Liu G. What is driving hospitals' patient-safety efforts? *Health Aff (Millwood)* 2004;23:103–115.

Rozovsky FA, Woods JR Jr, eds. *The Handbook of Patient Safety Compliance: A Practical Guide for Health Care Organizations.* San Francisco, CA: Jossey-Bass, 2005.

The Joint Commission. National Patient Safety Goals. Available at: http://www.jointcommission.org/PatientSafety/NationalPatientSafetyGoals/.

CHAPTER TWENTY ONE

The Role of Patients

OVERVIEW

With increasing public attention to patient safety came calls for more participation by patients and their advocates in the search for solutions. Some of these calls have focused on individual healthcare organizations, such as efforts to include patients on hospital safety committees.[1] Most of the calls for patient engagement, though, have involved enlisting patients in efforts to improve their own individual safety—often framed as a version of the question: "What can patients do to protect themselves?" This chapter will explore some of the opportunities and challenges surrounding patient engagement in their own safety.

LANGUAGE BARRIERS AND HEALTH LITERACY

A previously healthy 10-month-old girl was taken to a pediatrician's office by her monolingual Spanish-speaking parents when they noted their daughter's generalized weakness. The infant was diagnosed with iron-deficiency anemia. At the time of the clinic visit, there were no Spanish-speaking staff or interpreters available. One of the nurses spoke broken Spanish and in general terms was able to explain that the girl had "low blood" and needed to take a medication. The parents nodded in understanding. The pediatrician wrote the following prescription in English:

Fer-Gen-Sol iron, 15 mg per 0.6 mL, 1.2 mL daily (3.5 mg/kg)

The parents took the prescription to the pharmacy. The local pharmacy did not have a Spanish-speaking pharmacist on staff, nor did they obtain an interpreter. The pharmacist attempted to demonstrate proper dosing and administration using the medication dropper and the parents nodded their understanding. The prescription label on the bottle was written in English.

The parents administered the medication at home and, within 15 minutes, the 10-month-old vomited twice and appeared ill. They took her to the nearest emergency department, where the serum iron level 1 hour after ingestion was found to be 365 mcg/dL, two times the upper therapeutic limit. She was admitted to the hospital for intravenous hydration and observation. On questioning, the parents stated that they had given their child a tablespoon of the medication, a 12.5-fold overdose. Luckily, the baby rapidly improved and was discharged the next day.[2]

Any discussion of patient engagement needs to start from Square One— do patients understand their care and the benefits and risks of various diagnostic and therapeutic strategies? If patients cannot understand the basics of their clinical care, it seems unlikely that they can advocate for themselves when it comes to safety practices.

Unfortunately, many patients are in no position to understand even the basics of their care, let along to serve as bulwarks against errors. First of all, nearly 50 million Americans (15% of the population) speak a primary language other than English at home, and 22 million have limited English proficiency.[3] Both of these populations nearly doubled in the United States between 1980 and 2000 (Figure 21–1). Few hospitals have adequate translation services[4]—translation frequently takes place on an ad hoc basis, often by untrained clerical personnel or even family members. In one case, an 11-year-old sibling interpreter committed 58 interpretation errors, 84% of which had potential clinical consequences.[5] Recognizing this problem, California has introduced legislation to ban children from being asked to interpret for their family members.

Even when patients do speak English well, recent evidence has demonstrated the high prevalence of *low health literacy*. Health literacy is defined as "the degree to which individuals have the capacity to obtain, process, and understand basic health information and services needed to make appropriate health decisions."[6] It includes the skills that patients need to communicate with providers, read medical information, make decisions about treatments, carry out care regimens, and decide when and how to seek help. Studies have shown that nearly half of American

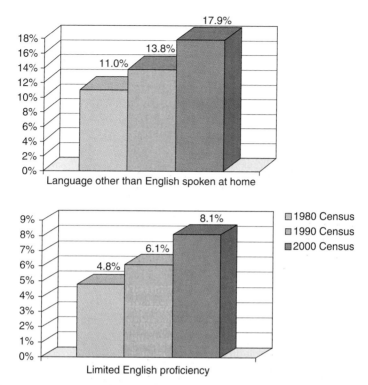

FIGURE 21–1.   Growth in U.S. populations (adults and children over age 4) who speak languages other than English at home, or who have limited English proficiency. (Reproduced with permission from U.S. Census Bureau data.)

adults have limited health literacy (Figure 21–2); the problems are greater in patients with lower income, less education, and lower English language proficiency. Low health literacy is associated with poor health-care outcomes.[7]

A number of strategies have been employed to mitigate the effect of low health literacy. Early efforts focused on identifying patients with low literacy,[8,9] and providing them with simplified health materials (such as brochures and medication labels), web sites, and interactive videos to help guide them to the right care. Newer interventions focus on training providers to interact with low health literacy patients in appropriate ways. For example, the use of the "teach back" (patients are asked to restate to the provider their understanding of their condition or treatment plan) can help ensure that patients truly comprehend their situation[10] (Figure 21–3). An alternative strategy is the "Ask Me 3," which prompts patients to ask their providers three questions: What is my main problem? What do I need to do? Why is it

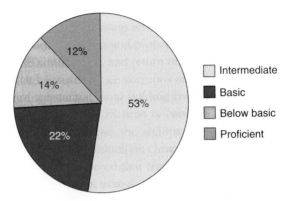

FIGURE 21–2. Health literacy of adults in the United States. Below Basic: circle date on doctor's appointment slip. Basic: give two reasons a person with no symptoms should get tested for cancer based on a clearly written pamphlet. Intermediate: determine what time to take Rx medicine based on label. Proficient: calculate employee share of health insurance costs using table. (Reproduced with permission from National Assessment of Adult Literacy, National Center for Educational Statistics, U.S. Department of Education, 2003.)

important for me to do this?[11] Patients who appear not to understand their care plan receive additional discussions and interventions.

In addition to these targeted interventions focused on the point of care, it will be important to integrate improved education about health literacy in the training of physicians, nurses, and pharmacists. For example, many of the

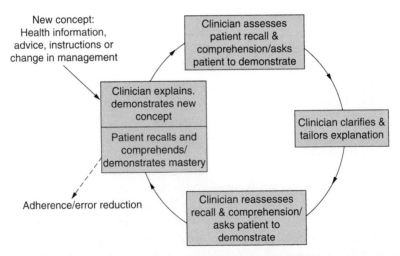

FIGURE 21–3. Example of a "teach back." (Reproduced with permission from Schillinger D, Piette J, Grumbach K, et al. Closing the loop: physician communication with diabetic patients who have low health literacy. *Arch Intern Med* 2003;163:83–90.)

newer competencies for residents involve issues of doctor-patient communication and improving physicians' sensitivity to patients varying communication styles and needs. Because many of the problems surrounding health literacy revolve around medications,[12] the involvement of trained pharmacists can be crucial.[13]

How do the issues of low English proficiency and poor health literacy impact patient safety? First of all, as in the case above, patients and families with problems in these areas are more likely to follow the wrong plan (such as taking the wrong medicine or using the wrong route of administration). Moreover, because patients are often too ashamed to admit that they don't understand the plan, caregivers may be unaware of their patients' limitations, in essence rendering ineffective any protection that might otherwise come through informed consent or patient vigilance.

"WHAT CAN PATIENTS DO TO PROTECT THEMSELVES?"

Obviously, the patient who does not speak English (or whatever the dominant language is) or who has poor health literacy is in no position to advocate for his or her own safety, nor to participate meaningfully in clinical decision-making and informed consent. This is a problem that needs to be tackled on its own merits.

But what about the patient who *is* competent and engaged, or who brings a family member to the clinical encounter who is able and willing to play an advocacy role? There are a number of questions that patients and families can ask to decrease their chances of becoming a victim of a medical error—some are shown in Appendix VII. Several advocacy groups and professional organizations have launched campaigns around this issue (e.g., the Joint Commission's "Speak up" campaign) (Table 21–1).[14]

However, as any healthcare provider who has been ill or has had a sick family member can attest, there are limits to what a layperson can do to protect him- or herself from medical mistakes. These limitations were pointed out most vividly by Dr. Don Berwick, the president of the Institute for Healthcare Improvement. Berwick's poignant tale of his wife's series of hospitalizations (at several Harvard hospitals) for an obscure neurologic disease demonstrates the limitations of depending on patients or their families—even those with highly informed and engaged family members— to prevent medical errors:

TABLE 21-1

The Joint Commission's "Speak Up" campaign

Speak up if you have questions or concerns, and if you don't understand, ask again. It's your body and you have a right to know.

Pay attention to the care you are receiving. Make sure you're getting the right treatments and medications by the right healthcare professionals. Don't assume anything.

Educate yourself about your diagnosis, the medical tests you are undergoing, and your treatment plan.

Ask a trusted family member or friend to be your advocate.

Know what medications you take and why you take them. Medication errors are the most common healthcare errors.

Use a hospital, clinic, surgery center, or other type of healthcare organization that has undergone a rigorous on-site evaluation against established state-of-the-art quality and safety standards, such as that provided by the Joint Commission.

Participate in all decisions about your treatment. You are the center of the healthcare team.

Reproduced with permission from www.jointcommission.org.

The errors were not rare; they were the norm. During one admission, the neurologist told us in the morning, "By no means should you be getting anticholinergic agents [a medication that can cause neurological and muscle changes]," and a medication with profound anticholinergic side effects was given that afternoon. The attending neurologist in another admission told us by phone that a crucial and potentially toxic drug should be started immediately. He said, "Time is of the essence." That was on Thursday morning at 10:00 am. The first dose was given 60 hours later—Saturday night at 10:00 p.m. Nothing I could do, nothing I did, nothing I could think of made any difference. It nearly drove me mad. Colace [a stool softener] was discontinued by a physician's order on Day 1, and was nonetheless brought by the nurse every single evening throughout a 14-day admission. Ann was supposed to receive five intravenous doses of a very toxic chemotherapy agent, but dose #3 was labeled as "dose #2." For half a day, no record could be found that dose #2 had ever been given, even though I had watched it drip in myself. I tell you from my personal observation, no day passed—not one—without a medication error.[15]

APOLOGIES: PHYSICIANS' AND HEALTHCARE SYSTEMS' OBLIGATIONS TO PATIENTS AND FAMILIES AFTER A MEDICAL ERROR

For generations, physicians and health systems responded with silence after a medical error. This was a natural outgrowth of the shame that most providers feel after an error (driven, in part, by the traditional view of errors as stemming from individual failures rather than system problems) and by a malpractice system that nurtures confrontation and leads providers to worry that an apology will be taken as an admission of guilt, only to be used against them later.

One of the most salutary aspects of the patient safety movement has been a rethinking of the role of apology. Many commentators, including some of the most influential figures in the field, have highlighted the ethical imperative to apologize to patients and families after errors.[16,17] A few U.S. states have passed legislation to prevent apologies from being used against physicians in malpractice suits. Training programs have begun to educate trainees about how to apologize (Table 21–2), having recognized that physicians' discomfort about their skills in this difficult task was one of the main obstacles,[18] and that physicians' and patients' views on what constitutes a meaningful apology are quite divergent.[19,20] Finally, some preliminary studies indicate that institutions that promote full disclosure to patients and families may lower their malpractice risk,[21] although some experts disagree.[22] A number of useful tools and monographs are now available to help teach caregivers how to apologize.[12,23–26] Some model language for telling a patient about a medication error is shown in Box 21–1.

TABLE 21–2

Four steps to full communication after a medical error

- Tell the patient and family what happened
- Take responsibility
- Apologize
- Explain what will be done to prevent future events

Reproduced with permission from Massachusetts Coalition for the Prevention of Medical Errors. *When Things Go Wrong: Responding to Adverse Events*. Available at: http://www. macoalition.org/documents/respondingToAdverseEvents.pdf.

BOX 21-1

MODEL LANGUAGE FOR TELLING A PATIENT ABOUT A MEDICATION ERROR

"Let me tell you what happened. We gave you a chemotherapeutic agent, carboplatin, instead of the pamidronate you were supposed to receive.

I want to discuss with you what this means for your health, but first I'd like to apologize.

I'm sorry. This shouldn't have happened. Right now, I don't know exactly how this happened, but I promise you that we're going to find out what happened and do everything we can to make sure that it doesn't happen again. I will share with you what we find as soon as I know, but it may take some time to get to the bottom of it all.

Once again, let me say how sorry I am that this happened.

Now, what does this mean for your health? You received only a fraction of the usual dose of carboplatin, so it is unlikely you will have any adverse effects from the infusion. However, I would like to monitor you closely over the next weeks. In patients who receive a full dose, the side effects we expect include . . . . We usually monitor patients for these side effects by . . . . We treat these side effects by . . . . I want to see you in my clinic tomorrow so we can . . . ."

Reproduced with permission from Massachusetts Coalition for the Prevention of Medical Errors. *When Things Go Wrong: Responding to Adverse Events.* Available at: http://www.macoalition.org/documents/respondingToAdverseEvents.pdf

---

PATIENT ENGAGEMENT AS A SAFETY STRATEGY

As Dr. Berwick's experience makes clear, there are real limitations on patients' abilities to protect themselves from medical errors. There are other potential problems as well. Although most providers welcome an informed patient or family member asking questions and being vigilant, some patients or families move from gentle inquiry into active conflict, forging a confrontational relationship with providers that might make them *less* safe. It would be human nature for a doctor or a nurse to think twice before entering such a patient's room—I have seen it happen.

More importantly, placing the onus for error prevention on patients or families risks displacing responsibility from providers, healthcare organizations, and policymakers. Why should it be a patient's responsibility to ensure that they don't receive the wrong medicine, or the wrong surgery? Or that providers wash their hands, or that handoffs are timely and accurate? When we step onto an airplane, we recognize that there is not much we can do to ensure our own safety—we simply trust that the airline and its employees have done everything they possibly can to keep us safe. A patient checking into a hospital or visiting a clinic or surgery center should be able to enjoy the same level of trust.

KEY POINTS

- Many patients have limited language proficiency and/or health literacy, which increases the risk that they will be victims of medical errors.

- Not only is an apology after a medical error the right thing to do, emerging evidence suggests that apologies do not increase, and may even decrease, malpractice risk.

- Patients and families can help participate in their own safety, but (a) there are limitations to this strategy's effectiveness, and (b) the responsibility to provide safe care should primarily be borne by providers, healthcare organizations, and policymakers, not patients.

REFERENCES

1. Conway JB, Weingart SN. Organizational change in the face of highly public errors I. The Dana-Farber Cancer Institute experience. AHRQ WebM&M (serial online), May 2005. Available at: http://www.webmm.ahrq.gov/perspective.aspx?perspectiveID=3.
2. Flores G. Language barrier. AHRQ WebM&M (serial online), April 2006. Available at: http://www.webmm.ahrq.gov/case.aspx?caseID=123.
3. U.S. Census Bureau. Selected social characteristics: 2004. Available at: http://factfinder.census.gov/servlet/ADPTable?_bm=y&-geo_id=01000US&-qr_name=ACS_2004_EST_G00_DP2&-ds_name= &-redoLog=false&-format.
4. Baker DW, Parker RM, Williams MV, et al. Use and effectiveness of interpreters in an emergency department. *JAMA* 1996;275:783–788.
5. Flores G, Laws MB, Mayo SJ, et al. Errors in medical interpretation and their potential clinical consequences in pediatric encounters. *Pediatrics* 2003;111:6–14.
6. Institute of Medicine. *Health Literacy: A Prescription to End Confusion.* Washington, DC: National Academy Press, 2004.
7. Literacy and Health Outcomes, Structured Abstract. Rockville, MD: Agency for Healthcare Research and Quality, January 2004. Available at: http://www.ahrq.gov/clinic/tp/littp.htm.
8. Davis TC, Long SW, Jackson RH, et al. Rapid estimate of adult literacy in medicine: a shortened screening instrument. *Fam Med* 1993;25: 391–395.

9. Parker RM, Baker DW, Williams MV, et al. The test of functional health literacy in adults: a new instrument for measuring patients' literacy skills. *J Gen Intern Med* 1995;10:537–541.

10. Schillinger D, Piette J, Grumbach K, et al. Closing the loop: physician communication with diabetic patients who have low health literacy. *Arch Intern Med* 2003;163:83–90.

11. Available at: http://www.p4chc.org.

12. Davis TC, Wolf MS, Bass PF III, et al. Literacy and misunderstanding prescription drug labels. *Ann Intern Med* 2006;145: 887–894.

13. Youmans SL, Schillinger D. Functional health literacy and medication use: the pharmacist's role. *Ann Pharmacother* 2003;37:1726–1729.

14. Available at: http://www.jointcommission.org.

15. Berwick DM. *Escape Fire: Lessons for the Future of Health Care*. New York, NY: The Commonwealth Fund, 2002.

16. Leape LL. Full disclosure and apology—an idea whose time has come. *Physician Exec* 2006;32:16–18.

17. Massachusetts Coalition for the Prevention of Medical Errors. *When Things Go Wrong: Responding to Adverse Events*. Available at: http://www. macoalition.org/documents/respondingToAdverseEvents.pdf.

18. Lazare A. Apology in medical practice: an emerging clinical skill. *JAMA* 2006;296:1401–1404.

19. Gallagher TH, Waterman AD, Ebers AG, et al. Patients' and physicians' attitudes regarding the disclosure of medical errors. *JAMA* 2003;289: 1001–1007.

20. Chan DK, Gallagher TH, Reznick R, et al. How surgeons disclose medical errors to patients: a study using standardized patients. *Surgery* 2005; 138:851–858.

21. Kachalia A, Shojania KG, Hofer TP, et al. Does full disclosure of medical errors affect malpractice liability? The jury is still out. *Jt Comm J Qual Saf* 2003;29:503–511.

22. Studdert DM, Mello MM, Gawande AA, et al. Disclosure of medical injury to patients: an improbable risk management strategy. *Health Aff (Millwood)* 2007;26:215–226.

23. Mazor KM, Simon SR, Gurwitz JH. Communicating with patients about medical errors: a review of the literature. *Arch Intern Med* 2004; 164:1690–1697.

24. Wu, AW. *Removing Insult from Injury: Disclosing Adverse Events*. Baltimore, MD: Johns Hopkins Bloomberg School of Public Health, 2005. Available at: http://www.jhsph.edu/dept/HPM/Research/Wu_video.html.

25. Anonymous. *Disclosing Medical Errors: A Guide to an Effective Explanation and Apology*. Oakbrook Terrace, IL: Joint Commission Resources, 2006.

26. Available at: http://www.sorryworks.net/.

ADDITIONAL READINGS

Flores G. Language barriers to health care in the United States. *N Engl J Med* 2006;355:229–231.

Karliner LS, Jacobs EA, Chen AH, et al. Do professional interpreters improve clinical care for patients with limited English proficiency? A systematic review of the literature. *Health Serv Res* 2007;42:727–754.

Lyons M. Should patients have a role in patient safety? A safety engineering view. *Qual Saf Health Care* 2007;16:140–142.

Marx D. Patient safety and the "just culture": a primer for health care executives. April 17, 2001. Available at: www.mers-tm.net/support/marx_primer.pdf.

Schillinger D. Misunderstanding prescription labels: the genie is out of the bottle. *Ann Intern Med* 2006;145:926–928.

Vincent CA, Coulter A. Patient safety: what about the patient? *Qual Saf Health Care* 2002;11:76–80.

Wu HW, Nishimi RY, Page-Lopez CM, et al. *Improving Patient Safety Through Informed Consent for Patients with Limited Health Literacy.* Washington, DC: National Quality Forum, 2005.

CHAPTER TWENTY TWO

Organizing a Safety Program

OVERVIEW

As the pressure to improve patient safety has grown, healthcare organizations, particularly hospitals but also larger healthcare systems, have struggled to create effective structures for their safety efforts. Although there are few data that allow comparisons between various organizational structures, best practices for promoting organizational safety have begun to emerge.[1–3] This chapter will explore some of these issues.

STRUCTURE AND FUNCTION

Before the year 2000, few organizations had patient safety committees or officers. Prior to that time, if there was any institutional focus on safety at all (in most institutions, there wasn't), it generally lived under the organization's top physician (sometimes a Vice President for Medical Affairs or Chief Medical Officer, or perhaps the elected Chief of the Medical Staff) or nurse (Chief Nursing Officer). In academic medical centers, safety issues may have been handled through the academic departmental structure (e.g., chair of the department of medicine or surgery), promoting a fragmented, siloed approach. When an institutional nonphysician leader did become involved in safety issues, it was usually a hospital risk manager, whose primary role was to protect the institution from liability. Although many risk managers considered preventing future errors to be part of their role, they rarely had the institutional clout or resources to make durable changes in processes, information technology, or culture. Larger institutions with quality committees or quality officers sometimes subsumed patient safety under these individuals or groups.

The latter structure is still common in small institutions that lack the resources to have independent safety operations, but many larger institutions have recognized the value of a separate organizational structure and group of personnel to focus on safety. The responsibilities of safety personnel include: monitoring and reacting to the incident reporting system, educating providers and others about new practices in safety (driven by the experience of others and the literature), measuring safety outcomes and developing programs to improve them, and supervising the approach to sentinel events (e.g., organizing root cause analyses) and to preventing future errors (e.g., carrying out Failure Mode Effects Analyses) (Chapter 14). In addition, such personnel must work collaboratively with other departments and personnel, such as those in information technology, quality, compliance, and risk management (see "Managing the Incident Reporting System," below).

MANAGING THE INCIDENT REPORTING SYSTEM

An organization interested in improving the quality of care (as opposed to patient safety) might not spend a huge amount of time and effort promoting reporting by caregivers to central administration. Why? To the extent that the quality issues of interest are measurable through outcome (mortality rates in patients with acute myocardial infarction, postoperative infection rates, readmission rates for patients with pneumonia) or process measures (Did every appropriate patient with myocardial infarction receive a beta-blocker and aspirin?) (Chapter 3), performance assessment does not depend on the direct involvement of the nurses and the doctors. Instead, these data can be collected through chart review or, increasingly, by tapping into electronic data streams created in the course of care. Obviously, when a quality leader identifies a "hot spot" through these measures, he or she cannot proceed without convening the relevant personnel to develop a complete understanding of the process and an action plan, but collecting the data can often be accomplished without provider participation.

Safety is different. In most cases, a Safety or Chief Medical Officer will have no way of discovering errors or risky situations without receiving this information from frontline workers. Although other mechanisms (direct observation of practice, trigger tools) can identify some problems, in most cases the providers are the repository of the knowledge needed to understand safety hazards, near misses, and true errors;

and thus to create the system changes to prevent them. As described in Chapter 14, the institutional incident reporting system is the usual vehicle for tapping into this rich vein of experience.

The *Patient Safety Officer* will generally be charged with managing the incident reporting system. At small institutions, he or she will likely review every report, aggregate the data into meaningful categories (e.g., medication errors, falls), and triage the reports for further action. Some reports will be simply noted, others will generate some analysis or an inquiry to a frontline manager, while still others will lead to a full blown root cause analysis (RCA). Many larger institutions have subdivided this task, selecting "category managers" to review the incidents in a given domain (a pharmacist for medication errors, a nurse-leader for falls, the Chief Medical Officer for reports of unprofessional physician behavior; Table 14–2). The category managers are expected to review data within their categories, take appropriate action, and triage cases to the safety officer (or even someone higher in the organization) when the error is particularly serious.

As with much of patient safety, results and culture are more important than structure. A technologically sophisticated incident reporting system will create little value if the frontline workers feel that the approach to reports is overly punitive, or if they see no evidence that reports are taken seriously or generate action (Chapter 15). So the safety officer will be well advised to spend as much time and energy making clear to providers that their reports lead to important changes as he or she does on purchasing and maintaining the system or producing sophisticated pie charts from it for other senior leaders.

DEALING WITH DATA

Although the safety officer will generally not be as data driven as the quality officer (for reasons described above), he or she will have a steady stream of inputs that can be important sources of understanding and action (Table 1–2). Some of these will be generated by the incident reporting system (see "Managing the Incident Reporting System," above); here, it is important to use the information effectively, while recognizing that voluntary reports only capture a small (and nonrandom) subset of errors and problems.[4] Malpractice claims are an even more serendipitous source of safety concerns (Chapter 18). For safety problems that can be measured as rates (such as hospital-acquired infections, Chapter 10), the role of the safety officer (assuming this is his domain; in large institutions, an infection control officer may be charged with this issue) becomes more like the quality officer: studying the data to see when rates have spiked above prior baselines or above local, regional, or national norms ("benchmarks"). In these circumstances, the safety officer will complete an in-depth analysis of the problem and develop an action plan to improve the outcomes. Increasingly, safety officers will need to audit areas that have been the subject of regulatory requirements or new institutional policies. Such audits are best done through direct observation, and recidivism should be expected. In fact, the safety officer should be worried if an audit 6 months after implementation of a new policy demonstrates 100% compliance with the practice: there is a good chance that these are biased data and more should be done to get a true snapshot of what is really happening. Finally, as medical records become electronic (Chapter 13), implementing innovative methods to screen caregiver notes, lab results and medication orders (such as via trigger tools, Chapter 14), and discharge summaries[5-7] will generate new and useful safety information.

One of the most important pieces of safety data will be the results of surveys of patient safety culture. There are several well-constructed, validated surveys that can be used for this purpose; a few have been used at enough institutions that results can be compared with those from like institutions or units (e.g., other academic medical centers, or other intensive care units [ICU]).[8] As discussed in Chapter 15, although it is intuitively appealing to think of institutions (such as hospitals or large healthcare delivery systems) as having organization-wide safety cultures, work by Sexton and others has demonstrated that safety culture tends to be local: even within a single hospital, there will be huge variations in culture between units down the hall from each other![9] The safety officer's job, then, is to ensure administration of the surveys and a reasonable response rate, that the results are thoughtfully analyzed, and—as always—that the data are converted into meaningful action. For clinical units with poor safety culture, it is critical to determine the nature of the problem. Is it poor leadership (if so, is leadership training or a new leader required)? Poor teamwork (should we consider a Crew Resource Management or other teamwork training program; Chapter 15)? And is there something to be learned from units with excellent culture that can be used to catalyze change in the more problematic units?[10]

STRATEGIES TO CONNECT SENIOR LEADERSHIP WITH FRONTLINE PERSONNEL

Recognizing that an effective safety program depends on connecting the senior leadership (who control major resources and policies) with what is truly happening on the clinical units, and further recognizing that incident reporting systems paint a very incomplete picture of this front line activity, many safety leaders have developed strategies to connect senior leadership with frontline caregivers. Two primary strategies have been promoted: Executive Walk Rounds and "Adopt-a-Unit."

Executive Walk Rounds is the healthcare version of the old business leadership strategy of MBWA ("Managing by Walking Around").[11–14] At some interval (some institutions do Walk Rounds weekly, others monthly), the safety officer will generally accompany another member of the senior leadership team (e.g., CEO, COO) to a unit in the institution—a medical floor, the emergency department, the labor and delivery suite, or perhaps an operating room. The visits are usually preannounced. Although the unit manager is generally present for the visit, the most important outcome is a frank discussion (with senior leadership spending more time listening than talking) about the problems and errors on the unit, and brainstorming solutions to these problems. Some institutions have formalized these visits with a script; a sample one is shown in Box 22–1.

Another strategy (not mutually exclusive, but institutions tend favor one or the other) is *"Adopt-a-Unit."*[15] Here, rather than executives visiting a wide variety of clinical areas around the hospital to get a broad picture of safety problems and issues, one senior leader adopts a given unit and attends relevant meetings with staff there (perhaps monthly) for a long period (6–12 months). This method, pioneered at Johns Hopkins, has the advantage of more sustained engagement and automatic follow-through, and the disadvantage of providing each leader a more narrow view of the entire institution. Given that there are only so many senior leaders to go around, the Adopt-a-Unit strategy will generally mean that certain units will be neglected. However, for the unit that is having important safety challenges or evidence of poor culture, this method, with its sustained focus, may have real value.

Whichever method is chosen, these efforts will be most useful if providers sense that senior leadership takes their concerns seriously, leaders demonstrate interest while being unafraid to show their ignorance about how

BOX 22–1

SELECTED SCRIPTS FOR PATIENT SAFETY EXECUTIVE WALK ROUNDS

Opening statements:

"We are moving as an organization to open communication and a blame-free environment because we believe that by doing so we can make your work environment safer for you and your patients."

"We're interested in focusing on the system and not individuals (no names are necessary)."

"The questions are very general, to help you think of areas to which the questions might apply consider medication errors, miscommunication between individuals (including arguments), distractions, inefficiencies, invasive treatments, falls, protocols not followed, and so on."

Questions to ask:

"Can you think of any events in the past day or few days that have resulted in prolonged hospitalization for a patient?"

Examples:

Appointments made but missed

Miscommunications

Delayed or omitted medications

"Have there been any near misses that almost caused patient harm but didn't?"

Examples:

Selecting a drug dose from the medications cart or pharmacy to administer to a patient and then realizing it's incorrect.

Misprogramming a pump, but having an alert warn you.

Incorrect orders by physicians or others caught by nurses or other staff.

"What aspects of the environment are likely to lead to the next patient harm?"

Examples:

Consider all aspects of admission, hospital stay, and discharge

Consider movement within the hospital

Consider communication

Consider informatics and computer issues

"Is there anything we could do to prevent the next adverse event?"

Examples:

What information would be helpful to you?

Consider alterations in the interaction between clinicians

Consider teamwork

Consider environment and workflow

"What specific intervention from leadership would make the work you do safer for patients?"

Examples:

Organize interdisciplinary groups to evaluate a specific problem.

Assist in changing the attitude of a particular group.

Facilitate interaction between two specific groups.

"How are we actively promoting a blame-free culture and working on the development of a blame-free reporting policy?"

Examples:

We do not penalize individuals for inadvertent errors.

The institution grants immunity to individuals who report adverse events in a timely fashion (where criminal behavior is not an issue).

Closing comment:

"We're going to work on the information you've given us. In return, we would like you to tell two other people you work with about the concepts we've discussed in this conversation."

Reproduced with permission from Frankel A. Patient Safety Leadership Walkrounds, Institute for Healthcare Improvement (IHI), 2004. Available at: http://www.wsha.org/files/82/WalkRounds1.pdf.

things really work on the floor, and the frontline workers later learn about how their input led to meaningful changes.

STRATEGIES TO GENERATE FRONT LINE ACTIVITY TO IMPROVE SAFETY

Although connecting providers to senior leadership is vitally important, units must also have the capacity to take action on their own. One of the dangers inherent in an organizational "safety program" will be that individual clinical units will not be sufficiently active and independent— sharing stories of errors, problem solving, and doing the daily work of making care safer. Because many such efforts do not require major changes in policies or large infusions of resources, safety officers and programs need to create an environment and culture in which such unit-based problem solving is the norm, not the exception.

While some units will instinctively move in this direction (often as a manifestation of strong local leadership and culture; Chapter 15), others will need help. Many of the programs discussed previously (such as Crew Resource Management training) should leave behind an ongoing organizational structure that supports unit-based safety. For example, at the University of California, San Francisco (UCSF), after more than 400 providers of all stripes participated in a healthcare Crew Resource Management program, we developed a unit-based safety team on our medical ward that collected stories, developed interdisciplinary case conferences, and convened periodically to problem solve on the unit. Their work was supported by e-CUSP, an electronic project management tool created for this purpose (Figure 22–1).[16, 17] This effort generated a new spirit of safety and problem solving on the unit, breathing life into many of the principles taught during the teamwork training.

Developing this kind of unit-based safety enterprise requires training, leadership, and some resources (perhaps a small amount of compensation for the unit-based champions, time for the group to meet, and food). It is also important to sort out the "cross-walk" between the unit-based efforts and the larger institutional safety program. On the one hand, the unit-based team must be free to discuss errors, develop educational materials, and problem solve without being encumbered by the organizational bureaucracy. On the other hand, the unit-based program cannot completely bypass the institutional incident reporting system, and it is vital that central leadership rapidly learns of major errors that should generate broader investigations, including root cause analyses.

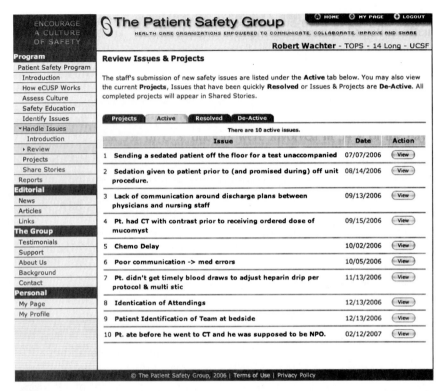

FIGURE 22–1. Screenshot from e-CUSP, a project management tool for unit-based safety programs. (Reproduced with permission from UCSF e-CUSP implementation of e-CUSP, The Patient Safety Group.)

DEALING WITH MAJOR ERRORS AND SENTINEL EVENTS

The process of a RCA is described in Chapter 14. The safety officer will often be charged with convening the RCA team, prepping senior leadership for the meetings, chairing the sessions, and converting the findings into a meaningful action plan. Because many states and the Joint Commission now either encourage or require that sentinel events (and the results of subsequent RCAs) are reported promptly, the safety officer has a key role in managing this process, often collaborating with the institutional risk manager if there are potential legal ramifications.

FAILURE MODE EFFECTS ANALYSES

The safety officer may also be charged with spearheading efforts to proactively assess and mitigate safety risks. The Joint Commission now requires that every organization carry out at least one Failure Mode Effects Analysis (FMEA) yearly. The process of and rationale behind FMEA is discussed in Chapter 14. Like the results of the RCA, the safety officer will often be responsible for converting the results of the FMEA into changes in policies and practice. In complex organizations, this requires tremendous diplomatic and organizational skill, because the changes often require approval by multiple committees and buy-in from a wide variety of stakeholders who may not have participated in the analysis and who lack a full understanding of patient safety or the issues at hand.

QUALIFICATIONS AND TRAINING OF THE PATIENT SAFETY OFFICER

The personal attributes of the patient safety officer are probably as important as his or her training and pedigree. Ideally, a safety officer will be a credible clinician with a strong interest in safety and specific training in many of the competencies described in the book: for example, human factors, information technology, data management, and culture change. He or she will be a team player—needing to constantly assemble and motivate interdisciplinary teams to problem solve. The officer will need to work collaboratively not only with frontline providers and senior leadership, but with armies of individuals with overlapping job descriptions: the quality officer, risk manager, information technology officer, compliance officer, and more. The larger the institution, the more likely that these functions will be managed by separate individuals. In smaller institutions, these hats (perhaps with the exception of the information technology officer) may all be worn by the same person!

THE ROLE OF THE PATIENT SAFETY COMMITTEE

Whether or not there is a designated patient safety officer, most institutions now have a patient safety committee, often a committee of the medical staff. This committee reviews adverse events and incident reports, helps to set and endorse safety-related policies, develops new safety initiatives, and disseminates information about patient safety to providers. In general, it will be made up of a diverse group of clinicians (physicians, nurses, pharmacists) and hospital administrators; a few institutions include lay members.

Patient safety committees need to address certain challenges. One is how the committee's activities will relate to those of other overlapping committees, such as risk management and quality improvement. This issue is parallel to the one the safety officer faces in interacting with his or her peers in these departments. And, like the safety officer, the correct answer involves combining appropriate amounts of overlap (some personnel should be shared across committees, so that each can know what the other is doing) with a clear mandate to focus on certain exclusive areas. A second issue is making sure that the committee reserves some time and energy to focus on issues that are not regulatory mandates. The committee that explicitly sets a goal of one to two group-generated projects per year is more likely to "think outside the box" than the group that spends all its time in reactive and compliance mode.

BOARD ENGAGEMENT IN PATIENT SAFETY

Up until recently, discussions about organizational leadership in safety tended to focus on the commitment and focus of the CEO and physician leaders. But in many healthcare organizations, the role of the board can be decisive in agenda setting and resource allocation.

Traditionally, hospital boards have delegated quality and safety to the medical staff, focusing instead on their fiduciary responsibilities. Why? Most board members are lay people (often prominent business and community leaders) who felt that they did (and perhaps could) not understand the clinical elements of quality and safety. Moreover, there were few useful measures to help boards understand the safety of their institutions.[18]

The safety movement has catapulted boards into action. Emerging evidence indicates that an engaged board can help promote safety, particularly when the board spends more than a quarter of its time on safety and quality issues, the board follows quality and safety data, senior executives are incentivized based on quality and safety, and there is active dialogue between the board and the medical staff.[19–21] The Institute for Healthcare Improvement's 5 Million Lives Campaign suggests a number of activities to promote board engagement in patient safety (Table 22–1).

TABLE 22–1

Six activities that boards should focus on to promote patient safety in their organizations

---

1. *Setting aims:* Set a specific aim to reduce harm this year. Make an explicit, public commitment to measurable quality improvement (e.g., reduction in unnecessary mortality and harm).

2. *Getting data and hearing stories:* Select and review progress toward safer care as the first agenda item at every board meeting. Put a "human face" on harm data.

3. *Establishing and monitoring system-level measures:* Identify a small group of organization-wide "roll-up" measures of patient safety (e.g., facility-wide harm, risk-adjusted mortality) that are continually updated and are made transparent to the entire organization and all of its customers.

4. *Changing the environment, policies, and culture:* Commit to establish and maintain an environment that is respectful, fair, and just for all who experience the pain and loss as a result of avoidable harm and adverse outcomes: the patients, their families, and the staff at the sharp end of error.

5. *Learning . . . Starting with the Board:* Develop your capability as a board. Learn about how "best in the world" boards work with executive and MD leaders to reduce harm. Set an expectation for similar levels of education and training for all staff.

6. *Establishing executive accountability:* Oversee the effective execution of a plan to achieve your aims to reduce harm including executive team accountability for clear quality improvement targets.

Reproduced with permission from Get Boards on Board How To Guide, Institute for Healthcare Improvement (IHI). Available at: http://www.ihi.org/IHI/Programs/Campaign/Campaign.htm?TabId=2.

RESEARCH IN PATIENT SAFETY

Until a decade ago, there was scant research in patient safety. At the time, a simplistic understanding of safety (as individual failings rather than systems problems) led to little interest in empirical investigation. After all, if an error is a screwup by an individual doctor or nurse, what exactly needs to be studied? This mindset led to little funding for patient safety research, few faculty who devoted their careers to it, and few journals interested in publishing the fruits of this research.

This has changed drastically over the past 10 years. In one small example, AHRQ (Agency for Healthcare Research and Quality) Patient Safety Network (a federal patient safety portal that I edit[22]) highlights 10–20 new research studies *every week* in the field of safety. The list of "Classic" articles, as defined by our editors and editorial board, now numbers more than 300.[23] Research funding for safety-oriented work is now more than 100 million dollars per year in the United States—largely from AHRQ, but also from other federal funders and a number of foundations. Scores of faculty have made patient safety research the focus of their professional careers, and many have been successful in garnering grants, publications, and promotion.

One of the exciting things about patient safety research is that it is inherently interdisciplinary and eclectic. Studies of medication errors, for example, often involve collaboration among physicians, nurses, pharmacists, and informatics experts. Studying errors at the man-machine interface may require engineers and human factors researchers. Studies of errors related to communication and poor teamwork may include psychologists and experts from other industries such as aviation.

Because patient safety involves real-world work processes, studies tend to be messier than controlled trials of new medications or laboratory studies of physiologic systems. It is very difficult to isolate the effect of one intervention (e.g., computerized provider order entry or Rapid Response Teams) from scores of other interventions occurring simultaneously.[24,25] It is nearly impossible to randomize hospital floors or institutions to one complex, expensive intervention or another, and thus institutions that embrace interventions often differ from those that don't in fundamental (and confounding) ways.

But young researchers should take heart—small studies that isolate the effect of a single intervention often lead to deeper understanding and catalyze larger research projects. For example, the simple matter of introducing "goal cards" to a clinical unit led to important improvements in communications and outcomes,[26,27] setting the stage for more ambitious teamwork and communication interventions. A study that randomized ICU residents to longer versus shorter shifts found far fewer errors in the latter group[28] and informed the debate over resident duty hours. Small studies demonstrated the value of several process changes in preventing catheter-related bloodstream infections,[29–31] ultimately leading to a multifaceted set of interventions that resulted in a remarkable dip in bloodstream infections in more than 100 ICUs.[32]

There is one more exciting aspect to patient safety research. In safety, unlike clinical medicine, the linkages to regulations, malpractice law, and media scrutiny can lead to rapid dissemination of "safety practices." For example, laws and regulations around nurse-to-patient ratios and medication reconciliation both came about after a relatively small number of studies demonstrated, or even hinted at, benefit. Because of this, well-designed and executed safety studies addressing important questions can rapidly lead to major changes in practice.

PATIENT SAFETY MEETS EVIDENCE-BASED MEDICINE

As research in safety has exploded, a fundamental question has arisen: what is the role of evidence in patient safety practices? There are two schools of thought on this. One group points out that many safety practices have little downside, have substantial face validity, and are too complex to study effectively and efficiently. For these reasons, they argue, traditional standards of evidence-based medicine should be relaxed for safety practices (such as Rapid Response Teams, computerized provider order entry, and teamwork training).[33] The other (which I tend to find myself more comfortable with) holds that safety practices often have unforeseen consequences, can be quite costly, and should be studied if possible (within reason, of course—few would argue that relatively inexpensive, easy, and commonsensical practices need to be rigorously studied before implementation)[25,34,35]. In our AHRQ evidence report, *Making Health Care Safer*, my colleagues and I came down this way on this crucial question:

> In the end, we are left with our feet firmly planted in the middle of competing paradigms. One argues that an evidence-based, scientific approach has served health care well and should not be relaxed simply because a popular practice from a "safer" industry sounds attractive. The other counters that medicine's slavish devotion to the scientific and epidemiologic method has placed us in a patient safety straightjacket, unable to consider the value of practices developed in other fields because of our myopic traditions and "reality."
>
> We see the merits in both arguments. Health care clearly has much to learn from other industries. Just as physicians must learn the "basic sciences" of immunology and molecular biology, providers and leaders interested in making health care safer must learn the "basic sciences" of organizational theory and human

factors engineering. Moreover, the "cases" presented on rounds should, in addition to classical clinical descriptions, also include the tragedy of the Challenger and the successes of Motorola. On the other hand, an unquestioning embrace of dozens of promising practices from other fields is likely to be wasteful, distracting, and potentially dangerous. We are drawn to a dictum from the Cold War era—"Trust, but verify."[36]

KEY POINTS

- Because of the intense focus on patient safety and increasing regulatory requirements, many organizations have begun safety programs, hired patient safety officers, and formed patient safety committees.

- The challenges of measuring safety mean that many of the inputs to safety programs will come from voluntary reporting, either through incident reporting systems or direct contacts between frontline personnel and safety leaders (such as via Executive Walk Rounds).

- Safety officers and programs need to effectively link with a variety of other personnel and programs: quality, risk management, information technology, and more.

- Safety research is difficult to do, but its results can be highly influential, particularly when they lead to regulatory action or other broad-based mandates.

- There is debate regarding the degree (if any) that traditional standards of evidence-based medicine should be relaxed for patient safety practices.

REFERENCES

1. In conversation with... Allan Frankel. AHRQ WebM&M (serial online), July 2006. Available at: http://webmm.ahrq.gov/perspective.aspx?perspective ID=26.
2. Whittington J. Key issues in developing a successful hospital safety program. AHRQ WebM&M (serial online), July 2006. Available at: http://webmm.ahrq.gov/perspective.aspx?perspectiveID=27.

3. Bagian JP, Lee C, Gosbee J, et al. Developing and deploying a patient safety program in a large health care delivery system: you can't fix what you don't know about. *Jt Comm J Qual Improv* 2001;27:522–532.

4. Cullen DJ, Bates DW, Small SD. Incident reporting system does not detect adverse drug events: a problem for quality improvement. *Jt Comm J Qual Improv* 1995;21:541–548.

5. Murff HJ, Forster AJ, Peterson JF, et al. Electronically screening discharge summaries for adverse medical events. *J Am Med Inform Assoc* 2003; 10:339–350.

6. Melton GB, Hripcsak G. Automated detection of adverse events using natural language processing of discharge summaries. *J Am Med Inform Assoc* 2005;12:448–457.

7. Forster AJ, Andrade J, van Walraven C. Validation of a discharge summary term search method to detect adverse events. *J Am Med Inform Assoc* 2005; 12:200–206.

8. Singla AK, Kitch BT, Weissman JS, et al. Assessing patient safety culture: a review and synthesis of the measurement tools. *J Patient Saf* 2006; 2:105–115.

9. Huang DT, Clermont G, Sexton JB, et al. Perceptions of safety culture vary across the intensive care units of a single institution. *Crit Care Med* 2007;35:165–176.

10. In conversation with... J. Bryan Sexton. AHRQ WebM&M (serial online), December 2006. Available at: http://www.webmm.ahrq.gov/perspective. aspx?perspectiveID=34.

11. Peters TJ, Waterman RJ. *In Search of Excellence: Lessons from America's Best Run Companies.* New York, NY: Collins, 2004.

12. Frankel A, Graydon-Baker E, Neppl C, et al. Patient safety leadership walkrounds. *Jt Comm J Qual Improv* 2003;29:16–26.

13. Frankel A, Grillo SP, Baker EG, et al. Patient safety leadership walkrounds at partners healthcare: learning from implementation. *Jt Comm J Qual Patient Saf* 2005;31:423–437.

14. Thomas EJ, Sexton JB, Neilands TB, et al. The effect of executive walk rounds on nurse safety climate attitudes: a randomized trial of clinical units. *BMC Health Serv Res* 2005;5:28.

15. Pronovost PJ. An interview with Peter Pronovost. *Jt Comm J Qual Saf* 2004;30:659–664.

16. Pronovost P, Weast B, Rosenstein B. Implementing and validating a comprehensive unit-based safety program. *J Patient Saf* 2005;1:33–40.

17. Pronovost P, King J, Holzmueller CG, et al. A web-based tool for the Comprehensive Unit-based Safety Program (CUSP). *J Comm J Qual Patient Saf* 2006;32:119–129.

18. In conversation with... Jim Reinertsen. AHRQ WebM&M (serial online), July 2007. Available at: http://webmm.ahrq.gov/perspective.aspx?perspective ID=45.

19. Joshi MS, Hines SC. Getting the board on board: engaging hospital boards in quality and patient safety. *Jt Comm J Qual Patient Saf* 2006;32:179–187.

20. Lockee C, Kroom K, Zablocki E, et al. *Quality.* San Diego, CA: The Governance Institute, 2006.

21. Kroch E, Vaughn T, Koepke M, et al. Hospital boards and quality dashboards. *J Patient Saf* 2006;2:10–19.

22. Available at: http://psnet.ahrq.gov.

23. Available at: http://psnet.ahrq.gov/classics.aspx.

24. Shojania KG, Duncan BW, McDonald KM, et al. Evidence-based review methodology. In: Shojania KG, Duncan BW, McDonald KM, et al., eds., *Making Health Care Safer: A Critical Analysis of Patient Safety Practices.* Evidence Report/Technology Assessment No. 43, AHRQ Publication No. 01-E058, July 2001.

25. Shojania KG. Interpreting the patient safety literature. AHRQ WebM&M (serial online), June 2005. Available at: http://webmm.ahrq.gov/perspective.aspx?perspectiveID=5.

26. Pronovost P, Berenholz S, Dorman T, et al. Improving communication in the ICU using daily goals. *J Crit Care* 2003;18:71–75.

27. Narasimhan M, Eisen LA, Mahoney CD, et al. Improving nurse-physician communication and satisfaction in the intensive care unit with a daily goals worksheet. *Am J Crit Care* 2006;15:217–222.

28. Landrigan CP, Rothschild JM, Cronin JW, et al. Effect of reducing interns' work hours on serious medical errors in intensive care units. *N Engl J Med* 2004;351:1838–1848.

29. Raad II, Hohn DC, Gilbreath BJ, et al. Prevention of central venous catheter-related infections by using maximal sterile barrier precautions during insertion. *Infect Control Hosp Epidemiol* 1994;15(4 Pt 1):231–238.

30. Chaiyakunapruk N, Veenstra DL, Lipsky BA, et al. Chlorhexidine compared with povidone-iodine solution for vascular catheter-site care: a meta-analysis. *Ann Intern Med* 2002;136:792–801.

31. Deshpande KS, Hatem C, Ulrich HL, et al. The incidence of infectious complications of central venous catheters at the subclavian, internal jugular, and femoral sites in an intensive care unit population. *Crit Care Med* 2005; 33:13–20; discussion 234–235.

32 Pronovost P, Needham D, Berenholtz S, et al. An intervention to decrease catheter-related bloodstream infections in the ICU. *N Engl J Med* 2006; 355:2725–2732.

33. Leape LL, Berwick DM, Bates DW. What practices will most improve safety? Evidence-based medicine meets patient safety. *JAMA* 2002; 288:501–507.

34. Shojania KG, Duncan BW, McDonald KM, et al. Safe but sound: patient safety meets evidence-based medicine. *JAMA* 2002;288:508–513.

35. Wachter RM. Expected and unanticipated consequences of the quality and information technology revolutions. *JAMA* 2006;295:2780–2783.

36. Shojania KG, Duncan BW, McDonald KM, et al. Drawing on safety practices from outside healthcare. In: Shojania KG, Duncan BW, McDonald KM, et al., eds., *Making Health Care Safer: A Critical Analysis of Patient Safety Practices*. Evidence Report/Technology Assessment No. 43, AHRQ Publication No. 01-E058, July 2001.

ADDITIONAL READINGS

Denham CR. Patient safety practices: leaders can turn barriers into accelerators. *J Patient Saf* 2005;1:41–55.

Denham CR. The new patient safety officer: a lifeline for patients, a life jacket for CEOs. *J Patient Saf* 2007;3:43–54.

Gandhi TK, Graydon-Baker E, Barnes JN, et al. Creating an integrated patient safety program. *Jt Comm J Qual Saf* 2003;29:383–390.

Gandhi TK, Graydon-Baker E, Neppl Huber C, et al. Closing the loop: follow-up and feedback in a patient safety program. *Jt Comm J Qual Patient Saf* 2005;31:614–621.

Rosen AB, Blendon RJ, DesRoches CM, et al. Physicians' views of interventions to reduce medical errors: does evidence of effectiveness matter? *Acad Med* 2005;80:189–192.

Rozovsky FA, Woods JR Jr, eds. *The Handbook of Patient Safety Compliance: A Practical Guide for Health Care Organizations*. San Francisco, CA: Jossey-Bass, 2005.

Conclusion

The fireworks that accompanied the publication of *To Err is Human* by the Institute of Medicine in late 1999 generated some magical thinking about how easy it would be to fix the problem of medical errors. A few computer systems here, some standard processes there (double checks, read backs), and maybe just a sprinkling of culture change—and poof, patients would be safer.

We now know how naïve this point of view was. The problem of medical errors is remarkably complex, and the solutions will need to be as varied as the problems. Do we need better information technology? Yes. Improved teamwork? Yes. Stronger rules and regulations? Yes. Training, simulation, decision support, forcing functions? Yes, yes, yes, and yes.

Organizationally, we have come to understand that solutions must be *both* top down and bottom up. Resources need to be made available from senior leadership and boards—for teamwork training, computers, and appropriate staffing. Yet much of the action in patient safety happens at the front line—will a nurse simply work around a hazardous situation, leaving it unfixed, or take the time and trouble to report it and help fix it? Will residents enthusiastically participate in teamwork training programs and M&M conferences? Will the senior surgeon welcome—truly welcome—input from the intern or the nurse who sees something that might put a patient at risk?

The analogies from other industries are extraordinarily helpful, but they take us only so far. Computerizing the hospital is far more challenging than computerizing the supermarket. Changing culture in the operating room is many times more complex than creating an environment in the hermetically sealed cockpit that allows two people—with similar training, expertise, and social status—to feel comfortable raising their concerns. Giving a patient a dozen medications safely is much more difficult than avoiding defects as a car slides down an assembly line. And yet there is much we can learn from all these settings, and that learning has truly begun.

And what is the proper role of patients in all of this? It is clear that patients should be involved in their care, and that patient engagement can be an important part of a comprehensive safety strategy. Moreover, being open and honest about our errors with patients and their families is undeniably right, independent of pragmatic considerations regarding whether such disclosures change the risk of a malpractice suit.

But why should a patient have to check into a hospital or enter a clinic and be worried—quite appropriately—that he or she will be injured by the medical system? We should be proud of the progress we have made in the relatively short time since the publication of *To Err is Human* by the Institute of Medicine jumpstarted the modern patient safety movement. But we cannot rest until patients can approach the healthcare system with the trepidation and anxiety borne of their illness and its possible sequelae, but free of fear that they will be harmed or killed in the process of being helped. We still have much to do before we get there.

Appendices

APPENDIX I. KEY BOOKS, REPORTS, SERIES, AND WEB SITES ON PATIENT SAFETY

*Key Books and Reports on Medical Errors and Errors More Generally**

1. Agency for Healthcare Research and Quality. *Advances in Patient Safety: From Research to Implementation.* Rockville, MD: Agency for Healthcare Research and Quality, February 2005. AHRQ Publication Nos. 050021 (1–4).
2. Banja J. *Medical Errors and Medical Narcissism.* Sudbury, MA: Jones and Bartlett Publishers, Inc., 2005.
3. Berwick DM. *Escape Fire: Designs for the Future of Health Care.* San Francisco, CA: Jossey-Bass, 2003.
4. Bogner MSE. *Human Error in Medicine.* Mahwah, NJ: Lawrence Erlbaum Associates, 1994.
5. Bosk CL. *Forgive and Remember: Managing Medical Failure,* 2nd ed. Chicago, IL: University of Chicago Press, 2003.
6. Casey SM. *Set Phasers on Stun: And Other True Tales of Design, Technology, and Human Error,* 2nd ed. Santa Barbara, CA: Aegean Publishing Company, 1998.
7. Cohen MR, ed. *Medication Errors,* 2nd ed. Washington, DC: American Pharmaceutical Association, 2006.
8. Columbia Accident Investigation Board. Report of the Columbia Accident Investigation Board, August 2003.
9. Donaldson L. An Organisation with a Memory: Report of an Expert Group on Learning from Adverse Events in the NHS Chaired by the Chief Medical Officer. London: The Stationery Office, 2000.

---

*Edited or written by Robert M. Wachter

10. Cook RI, Woods DD, Miller C. *A Tale of Two Stories: Contrasting Views of Patient Safety*. National Patient Safety Foundation at the AMA: Annenberg Center for Health Sciences, 1998.

11. Gawande A. *Complications: A Surgeon's Notes on an Imperfect Science*. New York, NY: Metropolitan Books, 2002.

12. Gawande A. *Better: A Surgeon's Notes on Performance*. New York, NY: Metropolitan Books, 2007.

13. Gibson R, Singh JP. *Wall of Silence: The Untold Story of the Medical Mistakes that Kill and Injure Millions of Americans*. Washington, DC: Lifeline, 2003.

14. Groopman J. *How Doctors Think*. Boston, MA: Houghton Mifflin, 2007.

15. Helmreich RL, Merritt AC. *Culture at Work in Aviation and Medicine: National, Organizational, and Professional Influences*. Aldershot, Hampshire, UK: Ashgate, 1998.

16. Kahneman D, Slovic P, Tversky A. *Judgment Under Uncertainty: Heuristics and Biases*. Cambridge, England: Cambridge University Press, 1987.

17. Massachusetts Coalition for the Prevention of Medical Errors. *When Things Go Wrong: Responding to Adverse Events*. Available at: http://www.macoalition.org/documents/respondingToAdverseEvents.pdf.

18. Merry A, Smith AM. *Errors, Medicine, and the Law*. Cambridge, England: Cambridge University Press, 2001.

19. Millenson ML. *Demanding Medical Excellence. Doctors and Accountability in the Information Age*. Chicago, IL: University of Chicago Press, 1997.

20. National Quality Forum. *Safe Practices for Better Healthcare. A Consensus Report*. Washington, DC: National Quality Forum, 2003.

21. Norman DA. *The Design of Everyday Things*. New York, NY: Basic Books, 2002.

22. Paget MA. *Unity of Mistakes: A Phenomenological Interpretation of Medical Work*. Philadelphia, PA: Temple University Press, 1993.

23. Paget MA. In: DeVault ML, ed., *Reflections on Cancer and an Abbreviated Life*. Philadelphia, PA: Temple University Press, 1993.

24. Perrow C. *Normal Accidents: Living with High-Risk Technologies. With a New Afterword and a Postscript on the Y2K Problem*. Princeton, NJ: Princeton University Press, 1999.

25. Reason JT. *Human Error*. New York, NY: Cambridge University Press, 1990.

26. Reason JT. *Managing the Risks of Organizational Accidents*. Aldershot, Hampshire, UK: Ashgate, 1997.

27. Robins NS. *The Girl who Died Twice: Every Patient's Nightmare: The Libby Zion Case and the Hidden Hazards of Hospitals*. New York, NY: Delacorte Press, 1995.

28. Rogers EM. *Diffusion of Innovation*, 5th ed. New York, NY: Free Press, 2003.
29. Rosenthal MM, Sutcliffe KM, eds. *Medical Error. What Do We Know? What Do We Do?* San Francisco, CA: John Wiley & Sons, 2002.
30. Rozovsky FA, Woods JR Jr, eds. *The Handbook of Patient Safety Compliance: A Practical Guide for Health Care Organizations.* San Francisco, CA: Jossey-Bass, 2005.
31. Sagan SD. *The Limits of Safety: Organizations, Accidents and Nuclear Weapons.* Princeton, NJ: Princeton University Press, 1993.
32. Scobie S, Thomson R. *Building a Memory: Preventing Harm, Reducing Risks and Improving Patient Safety.* London, England: National Patient Safety Agency, 2005.
33. Sharpe VA, Faden AI. *Medical Harm: Historical, Conceptual, and Ethical Dimensions of Iatrogenic Illness.* New York, NY: Cambridge University Press, 1998.
34. *Shojania KG, Duncan BW, McDonald KM, Wachter RM, eds. *Making Health Care Safer: A Critical Analysis of Patient Safety Practices.* Evidence Report/Technology Assessment No. 43 from the Agency for Healthcare Research and Quality: AHRQ Publication No. 01-E058, July 2001. Available at: http://www.ahrq.gov/clinic/ptsafety/.
35. Spath PL. *Error Reduction in Health Care: A Systems Approach to Improving Patient Safety.* San Francisco, CA: Jossey-Bass, 1999.
36. Stewart JB. *Blind Eye: How the Medical Establishment Let a Doctor Get Away with Murder.* New York, NY: Simon & Schuster, 1999.
37. Tenner E. *Why Things Bite Back: Technology and the Revenge of Unintended Consequences.* New York, NY: A. A. Knopf, 1996.
38. Vaughan D. *The Challenger Launch Decision: Risky Technology, Culture, and Deviance at NASA.* Chicago, IL: University of Chicago Press, 1997.
39. Vincent C. *Patient Safety.* London: Elsevier, 2005.
40. *Wachter RM, Shojania KG. *Internal Bleeding: The Truth Behind America's Terrifying Epidemic of Medical Mistakes.* New York, NY: Rugged Land, 2004.
41. Weick KE. *Sensemaking in Organizations.* Thousand Oaks, CA: Sage Publications, 1995.
42. Weick KE, Sutcliffe KM. *Managing the Unexpected: Assuring High Performance in an Age of Complexity.* San Francisco, CA: Jossey-Bass, 2001.
43 Wiener EL, Kanki BG, Helmreich RL. *Cockpit Resource Management.* San Diego, CA: Academic Press, 1993.
44. Wu HW, Nishimi RY, Page-Lopez CM, et al. *Improving Patient Safety Through Informed Consent for Patients with Limited Health Literacy.* Washington, DC: National Quality Forum, 2005.

The Institute of Medicine (IOM) Reports on Medical Errors and Healthcare Quality (The Quality Chasm Series)

1. Kohn L, Corrigan J, Donaldson M, eds. *To Err is Human: Building a Safer Health System.* Washington, DC: Committee on Quality of Health Care in America, Institute of Medicine: National Academy Press, 2000. ["The IOM Report"]
2. Committee on Quality of Health Care in America, IOM. *Crossing the Quality Chasm: A New Health System for the 21st Century.* Washington, DC: National Academy Press, 2001.
3. Page A, ed. *Keeping Patients Safe. Transforming the Work Environment of Nurses.* Committee on the Work Environment for Nurses and Patient Safety, Board on Health Care Services. Washington, DC: National Academy Press, 2004.
4. Aspden P, Corrigan JM, Wolcott J, et al. *Patient Safety: Achieving a New Standard for Care.* Washington, DC: National Academy Press, 2004.
5. Nielsen-Bohlman L, Panzer AM, Kindig DA. Institute of Medicine Committee on Health Literacy. *Health Literacy: A Prescription to End Confusion.* Washington, DC: National Academy Press, 2004.
6. Aspden P, Wolcott J, Bootman JL, et al., eds. *Preventing Medication Errors.* Committee on Identifying and Preventing Medication Errors. Washington, DC: National Academy Press, 2007.

Quality Grand Rounds Series, Annals of Internal Medicine*

1. *Wachter RM, Shojania KG, Saint S, et al. Learning from our mistakes: Quality Grand Rounds, a new case-based series on medical errors and patient safety. *Ann Intern Med* 2002;136:850–852.
2. Chassin MR, Becher EC. The wrong patient. *Ann Intern Med* 2002; 136:826–833.
3. Bates DW. Unexpected hypoglycemia in a critically ill patient. *Ann Intern Med* 2002;137:110–116.
4. Hofer TP, Hayward RA. Are bad outcomes from questionable clinical decisions preventable medical errors? A case of cascade iatrogenesis. *Ann Intern Med* 2002;137:327–333.
5. Gerberding JL. Hospital-onset infections: a patient safety issue. *Ann Intern Med* 2002;137:665–670.

---

*Edited or written by Robert M. Wachter

6. Cleary PD. A hospitalization from hell: a patient's perspective on quality. *Ann Intern Med* 2003;138:33–39.

7. Lynn J, Goldstein NE. Advance care planning for fatal chronic illness: avoiding commonplace errors and unwarranted suffering. *Ann Intern Med* 2003;138:812–818.

8. Brennan TA, Mello MM. Patient safety and medical malpractice: a case study. *Ann Intern Med* 2003;139:267–273.

9. Goldman L, Kirtane AJ. Triage of patients with acute chest pain and possible cardiac ischemia: the elusive search for diagnostic perfection. *Ann Intern Med* 2003;139:987–995.

10. Pronovost PJ, Wu AW, Sexton JB. Acute decompensation after removing a central line: practical approaches to increasing safety in the intensive care unit. *Ann Intern Med* 2004;140:1025–1033.

11. Redelmeier DA. Improving patient care. The cognitive psychology of missed diagnoses. *Ann Intern Med* 2005;142:115–120.

12. Gandhi TK. Fumbled hand-offs: one dropped ball after another. *Ann Intern Med* 2005;142:352–358.

13. McDonald CJ. Computerization can create safety hazards: a bar-coding near miss. *Ann Intern Med* 2006;144:510–516.

14. Shojania KG, Fletcher KE, Saint S. Graduate medical education and patient safety: a busy—and occasionally hazardous—intersection. *Ann Intern Med* 2006;145:592–598.

15. *Wachter RM, Shojania KG, Markowitz AJ, et al. Quality Grand Rounds: the case for patient safety. *Ann Intern Med* 2006;148:629–630.

*Web sites and Theme Issues on Medical Errors**

Agency for Healthcare Research and Quality (AHRQ): Medical Errors & Patient Safety. Available at: http://ahrq.gov/qual/errorsix.htm.

*AHRQ Patient Safety Network (PSNet). Available at: http://www.psnet.ahrq.gov.

*AHRQ WebM&M: Morbidity and Mortality Rounds on the Web. Available at: http://www.webmm.ahrq.gov/.

Theme issue on medical error. *BMJ* 2000;320(7237). Available at: http://bmj.com/content/vol320/issue7237/.

Theme issue on medical error. *Eff Clin Pract* 2000. Available at: http://www.acponline.org/journals/ecp/pastiss/nd00.htm.

FDA Patient Safety News. Available at: http://www.fda.gov/cdrh/psn.

Institute for Healthcare Improvement (IHI). Available at: http://www.ihi.org.

---

*Edited or written by Robert M. Wachter

Institute for Safe Medication Practices. Available at: http://www.ismp.org/.

Joint Commission. Available at: http://www.jointcommission.org.

Focus on computerized provider order systems. *J Am Med Inform Assoc* 2007;14:25–75. Available at: http://www.jamia.org/content/vol14/issue1/.

Leapfrog Group for Patient Safety. Available at: http://www.leapfroggroup.org/.

National Patient Safety Agency (United Kingdom). Available at: http://www.npsa.nhs.uk/.

National Patient Safety Foundation. Available at: http://www.npsf.org/.

National Quality Forum. Available at: http://www.qualityforum.org.

Profiles in Patient Safety. Case-based series of articles. *Acad Emerg Med.* Available at: http://www.aemj.org/cgi/content/full/9/4/324.

World Alliance for Patient Safety (World Health Organization). Available at: http://www.who.int/patientsafety/en/.

APPENDIX II. GLOSSARY OF SELECTED TERMS IN PATIENT SAFETY

Active error (or active failure)—Errors that occur at the point of contact between a human and some aspect of a larger system (e.g., a human-machine interface). They are generally readily apparent (e.g., pushing an incorrect button, ignoring a warning light) and almost always involve someone at the front line. Latent errors (or latent conditions), in contrast, refer to less apparent failures of organization or design that contributed to the occurrence of errors or allowed them to cause harm to patients.

Active failures are sometimes referred to as errors at the "sharp end," figuratively referring to a scalpel. In other words, errors at the sharp end are noticed first because they are committed by the person closest to the patient. This person may literally be holding a scalpel (e.g., an orthopedist who operates on the wrong leg) or figuratively be administering any kind of therapy (e.g., a nurse programming an intravenous pump). To complete the metaphor, latent errors are those at the other end of the scalpel—the "blunt end"—referring to the many layers of the healthcare system that affect the person "holding" the scalpel.

Adverse drug event (ADE)—An adverse event involving medication use. Examples are:

- Anaphylaxis to penicillin
- Major hemorrhage from heparin

- Aminoglycoside-induced renal failure
- Agranulocytosis from chloramphenicol

As with the more general term "adverse event", there is no necessary relation to error or poor quality of care. In other words, ADEs include expected adverse drug reactions ("side effects"), as well as events caused by error. Thus, a serious allergic reaction to penicillin in a patient with no prior such history is an ADE, but so is the same reaction in a patient who does have a known allergy history but receives penicillin as a result of a prescribing oversight (the latter is also an error).

Adverse event—Any injury caused by medical care. Examples are:

- Pneumothorax from central venous catheter placement
- Anaphylaxis to penicillin
- Postoperative wound infection
- Hospital-acquired delirium (or "sundowning") in elderly patients

Identifying something as an adverse event does not imply "error," "negligence," or poor quality care. It simply indicates that an undesirable clinical outcome resulted from some aspect of diagnosis or therapy, not an underlying disease process. Thus, pneumothorax from central venous catheter placement counts as an adverse event regardless of insertion technique. Similarly, postoperative wound infections count as adverse events even if the operation adhered to sterile procedures, the patient received appropriate antibiotic prophylaxis in the perioperative setting, and so on. See also "iatrogenic".

Anchoring error (or bias)—Refers to the common cognitive trap of allowing first impressions to exert undue influence on the diagnostic process. Clinicians often latch on to features of a patient's presentation that suggest a specific diagnosis. Often, this initial diagnostic impression will prove correct. However, in some cases, subsequent developments in the patient's course will prove inconsistent with the first impression. Anchoring bias refers to the tendency to hold on to the initial diagnosis, even in the face of disconfirming evidence.

Authority gradient—Refers to the balance of decision-making power or the steepness of command hierarchy in a given situation. Members of a crew or organization with a domineering, overbearing, or dictatorial team leader experience a steep authority gradient. Expressing concerns, questioning, or even simply clarifying instructions would require considerable determination on the part of team members who perceive their input as devalued or frankly unwelcome. Most teams require some degree of authority gradient; otherwise roles are blurred and decisions cannot be made in a timely fashion. However, effective team leaders consciously establish a command hierarchy appropriate to the training and experience of team members.

Availability bias (or heuristic)—Refers to the tendency to assume, when judging probabilities or predicting outcomes, that the first possibility that comes to mind (i.e., the most cognitively "available" possibility) is also the most likely possibility. For instance, suppose a patient presents with intermittent episodes of very high blood pressure. Because episodic hypertension resembles textbook descriptions of pheochromocytoma, a memorable but uncommon endocrinologic tumor, this diagnosis may immediately come to mind. A clinician who infers from this immediate association that pheochromocytoma is the most likely diagnosis would be exhibiting availability bias.

Bayesian approach—Probabilistic reasoning in which test results (not just laboratory investigations, but history, physical examination, or any aspect for the diagnostic process) are combined with prior beliefs about the probability of a particular disease. One way of recognizing the need for a Bayesian approach is to recognize the difference between the performance of a test in a population and in an individual. At the population level, we can say that a test has a sensitivity and specificity of, say, 90%—that is, 90% of patients with the condition of interest have a positive result and 90% of patients without the condition have a negative result. In practice, however, a clinician needs to attempt to predict whether an individual patient with a positive or negative result does or does not have the condition of interest. This prediction requires combining the observed test result not just with the known sensitivity and specificity, but also with an estimate of the chance the patient had the disease in the first place (based on demographic factors, findings on examination, or general clinical gestalt).

Benchmark—Refers to an attribute or achievement that serves as a standard for other providers or institutions to emulate. Benchmarks differ from other "standard of care" goals in that they derive from empiric data—specifically, performance or outcomes data. For example, a statewide survey might produce risk-adjusted 30-day rates for death or other major adverse outcomes. After adjusting for relevant clinical factors, the top 10% of hospitals can be identified in terms of particular outcome measures. These institutions would then provide benchmark data on these outcomes.

Blunt end—Refers to the many layers of the healthcare system not in direct contact with patients, but which influence the personnel and equipment at the "sharp end" who do contact patients. The blunt end thus consists of those who set policy, manage healthcare institutions, design medical devices, and other people and forces, which, though removed in time and space from direct patient care, nonetheless affect how care is delivered. Thus, an error programming an intravenous pump would represent a problem at the sharp end, while the institution's decision to use multiple different types of infusion pumps, making programming errors more likely, would represent a problem at the blunt end. The terminology of "sharp" and "blunt" ends corresponds roughly to "active failures" and "latent conditions."

Checklist—Algorithmic listing of actions to be performed in a given clinical setting (e.g., advanced cardiac life support [ACLS] protocols for treating cardiac arrest) to ensure that, no mater how often performed by a given practitioner, no step will be forgotten. An analogy is often made to flight preparation in aviation, as pilots and air traffic controllers follow pretakeoff checklists regardless of how many times they have carried out the tasks involved.

Clinical decision support system (CDSS)—Any system designed to improve clinical decision making related to diagnostic or therapeutic processes of care. CDSSs thus address activities ranging from the selection of drugs (e.g., the optimal antibiotic choice given specific microbiologic data) or diagnostic tests, to detailed support for optimal drug dosing and support for resolving diagnostic dilemmas. Structured antibiotic order forms represent a common example of paper-based CDSSs. Although such systems are still commonly encountered, many people now equate CDSSs with computerized systems in which software algorithms generate patient-specific recommendations by matching characteristics, such as age, renal function, or allergy history, with rules in a computerized knowledge base. The distinction between decision support and simple reminders can be unclear, but usually reminder systems are included as decision support if they involve patient-specific information. For instance, a generic reminder (e.g., "Did you obtain an allergy history?") would not be considered decision support, but a warning (e.g., "This patient is allergic to codeine.") that appears at the time of entering an order for codeine would be. See also "computerized provider order entry."

Close call—An event or situation that did not produce patient injury, but only because of chance. This good fortune might reflect robustness of the patient (e.g., a patient with penicillin allergy receives penicillin, but has no reaction) or a fortuitous, timely intervention (e.g., a nurse happens to realize that a physician wrote an order in the wrong chart). Such events have also been termed "near-miss" incidents.

Competency—Having the necessary knowledge or technical skill to perform a given procedure within the bounds of success and failure rates deemed compatible with acceptable care.

Computerized provider order entry or computerized physician order entry (CPOE)—Refers to a computer-based system of ordering medications and often other tests. Physicians (or other providers) directly enter orders into a computer system that can have varying levels of sophistication. Basic CPOE ensures standardized, legible, complete orders, and thus primarily reduces errors caused by poor handwriting and ambiguous abbreviations. Almost all CPOE systems offer some additional capabilities, which fall under the general rubric of CDSS. Typical CDSS features involve suggested default values for drug doses, routes of administration, or frequency. More sophisticated CDSSs can perform drug allergy checks (e.g., the user orders ceftriaxone and a warning flashes that the patient has a documented penicillin allergy), drug-laboratory value checks (e.g., initiating an order for gentamicin prompts the system to alert you to the patient's last creatinine), drug-drug interaction checks, and so on. At the highest level of sophistication, CDSS prevents not only errors of commission (e.g., ordering a drug in excessive doses or in the setting of a serious allergy), but also of omission. For example, an alert may appear such as, "You have ordered heparin; would you like to order a partial thromboplastin time (PTT) in 6 hours?" Or, even more sophisticated: "The admitting diagnosis is hip fracture; would you like to order heparin for deep vein thrombosis (DVT) prophylaxis?" See also "clinical decision support system."

Confirmation bias—Refers to the tendency to focus on evidence that supports a working hypothesis, such as a diagnosis in clinical medicine, rather than to look for evidence that refutes it or provides greater support to an alternative diagnosis. Suppose a 65-year-old man with a past history of angina presents to the emergency department with acute onset of shortness of breath. The physician immediately considers the possibility of cardiac ischemia, so asks the patient if he has experienced any chest pain. The patient replies affirmatively. Because the physician perceives this answer as confirming his working diagnosis, he does not ask if the chest pain was pleuritic in nature, which would decrease the likelihood of an acute coronary syndrome and increase the likelihood of pulmonary embolism, a reasonable alternative diagnosis. In many cases, especially in acute care medicine, clinicians have the results of numerous tests in hand when they first meet a patient. The results of these tests often do not all suggest the same diagnosis. The appeal of accentuating confirmatory test results and ignoring nonconfirmatory ones is that it minimizes cognitive dissonance. A related cognitive trap that may accompany confirmation bias and compound the possibility of error is "anchoring bias"—the tendency to stick with one's first impressions, even in the face of significant disconfirming evidence. See also "anchoring bias."

Crew Resource Management (CRM)—Also called Crisis Resource Management in some contexts (e.g., anesthesia), encompasses a range of approaches to training groups to function as teams, rather than as collections of individuals. Originally developed in aviation, CRM emphasizes the role of "human factors"—the effects of fatigue, expected or predictable perceptual errors (such as misreading monitors or mishearing instructions), as well as the impact of different management styles and organizational cultures in high-stress, high-risk environments. CRM training develops communication skills, fosters a more cohesive environment among team members, and creates an atmosphere in which junior personnel will feel free to speak up when they think that something is amiss. Some CRM programs emphasize education on the settings in which errors occur and the aspects of team decision making conducive to "trapping" errors before they cause harm. Other programs provide more hands-on training involving simulated crisis scenarios followed by debriefing sessions in which participants assess their own and others' behavior.

Critical incidents—Jeffrey Cooper and colleagues defined critical incidents as occurrences that are "significant or pivotal, in either a desirable or an undesirable way." This definition by itself conveys little—what does "significant or pivotal" mean? In many ways, it is the spirit of the expression in quality improvement circles, "every defect is a treasure." In other words, these incidents, whether close calls or disasters in which significant harm occurred, provide valuable opportunities to learn about individual and organizational factors that can be remedied to prevent similar incidents in the future.

Decision support—Refers to any system for advising or providing guidance about a particular clinical decision at the point of care. For example, a copy of an algorithm for antibiotic selection in patients with community-acquired pneumonia would count as clinical decision support if made available at the point of care. Increasingly, decision support occurs via a computerized clinical information or order entry system. Typically, a decision support system responds to "triggers" or "flags"—specific diagnoses, laboratory results, medication choices, or complex combinations of such parameters—and provides information or recommendations directly relevant to a specific patient encounter. For instance, ordering an aminoglycoside for a patient with creatinine above a certain value might trigger a message suggesting a dose adjustment. See also "clinical decision support system."

Error—An act of commission (doing something wrong) or omission (failing to do the right thing) that leads to an undesirable outcome or significant potential for such an outcome. For instance, ordering a medication for a patient with a documented allergy to that medication would be an act of commission. Failing to prescribe a proven medication with major benefits for an eligible patient (e.g., low-dose heparin as venous thromboembolism prophylaxis for a patient after hip replacement surgery) would represent an error of omission. Errors of omission are more difficult to recognize than errors of commission but likely represent a larger problem.

Error chain—Refers to the series of events that led to a disastrous outcome, typically uncovered by a root cause analysis (RCA). Sometimes the chain metaphor carries the added sense of inexorability, as many of the causes are tightly coupled, such that one problem begets the next. A more specific meaning of error chain, especially when used in the phrase "break the error chain," relates to the common themes or categories of causes that emerge from root cause analyses. These categories generally include (1) failure to follow standard operating procedures, (2) poor leadership, (3) breakdowns in communication or teamwork, (4) overlooking or ignoring individual fallibility, and (5) losing track of objectives. Used in this way, break the error chain is shorthand for an approach in which team members continually address these links as a crisis or routine situation unfolds. The checklists that are included in teamwork training programs have categories corresponding to these common links in the error chain (e.g., establish team leader, assign roles and responsibilities, monitor your teammates).

Face validity—The extent to which a technical concept, instrument, or study result is plausible, usually because its findings are consistent with prior assumptions and expectations.

Failure mode and effects analysis (FMEA)—Error analysis may involve retrospective investigations (as in RCA) or prospective attempts to predict "error modes." One commonly used approach for the latter is FMEA, in which the likelihood of a particular process failure is combined with an estimate of the relative impact of that error to produce a "criticality index." By combining the probability of failure with the consequences of failure, this index allows for the prioritization of specific processes as quality improvement targets.

Failure to rescue—Shorthand for failure to rescue (i.e., prevent a clinically important deterioration, such as death or permanent disability) from a complication of an underlying illness (e.g., cardiac arrest in a patient with acute myocardial infarction) or a complication of medical care (e.g., major hemorrhage after thrombolysis for acute myocardial infarction). Failure to rescue thus provides a measure of the degree to which providers responded to adverse occurrences (e.g., hospital-acquired infections, cardiac arrest or shock) that developed on their watch. It may reflect the quality of monitoring, the effectiveness of actions taken once early complications are recognized, or both.

Forcing function—An aspect of a design that prevents a target action from being performed or allows its performance only if another specific action is performed first. For example, automobiles are now designed so that the driver cannot shift into reverse without first putting his or her foot on the brake pedal. Forcing functions need not involve device design. For instance, one of the first forcing functions identified in healthcare was the removal of concentrated potassium from general hospital wards.

Health literacy—Individuals' ability to find, process, and comprehend the basic health information necessary to act on medical instructions and make decisions about their health.

Heuristic—Loosely defined or informal rule often arrived at through experience or trial and error (e.g., gastrointestinal complaints that wake patients up at night are unlikely to be functional). Heuristics provide cognitive shortcuts in the face of complex situations, and thus serve an important purpose. Unfortunately, they can also turn out to be wrong.

The Health Insurance Portability and Accountability Act (HIPAA)—The 1996 federal regulations intended to increase privacy and security of patient information during electronic transmission or communication of "protected health information" (PHI) among providers or between providers and payers or other entities.

High reliability organizations (HROs)—Organizations or systems that operate in hazardous conditions but have fewer than their fair share of adverse events. Commonly discussed examples include air traffic control systems, nuclear power plants, and naval aircraft carriers. Detailed case studies of specific HROs have identified some common features, which have been offered as models for other organizations to achieve substantial improvements in their safety records. These features include:

- Preoccupation with failure—the acknowledgment of the high-risk, error-prone nature of an organization's activities and the determination to achieve consistently safe operations.

- Commitment to resilience—the development of capacities to detect unexpected threats and contain them before they cause harm, or bounce back when they do.

- Sensitivity to operations—attentiveness to the issues facing workers at the front line. Management units at the front line are given some autonomy in identifying and responding to threats, rather than adopting a rigid top-down approach.

- A culture of safety, in which individuals feel comfortable drawing attention to potential hazards or actual failures without fear of censure from management.

Hindsight bias—In a very general sense, hindsight bias relates to the common expression "hindsight is 20/20." This expression captures the tendency for people to regard past events as expected or obvious, even when, in real time, the events perplexed those involved. In the context of safety analysis, hindsight bias refers to the tendency to judge the events leading up to an accident as errors because the bad outcome is known. The more severe the outcome, the more likely that decisions leading up to this outcome will be judged as errors.

Human factors (or human factors engineering)—Refers to the study of human abilities and characteristics as they affect the design and smooth operation of equipment, systems, and jobs. The field concerns itself with considerations of the strengths and weaknesses of human physical and mental abilities and how these affect the systems design. Human factors analysis does not require designing or redesigning existing objects. For instance, the now generally accepted recommendation that hospitals standardize equipment such as ventilators, programmable IV pumps, and defibrillators (i.e., that each hospital picks a single type, so that different floors do not have different defibrillators) is an example of a very basic application of a heuristic from human factors that equipment be standardized within a system wherever possible.

Iatrogenic—An adverse effect of medical care, rather than of the underlying disease (literally "brought forth by healer," from Greek iatros, for healer, and gennan, to bring forth); equivalent to adverse event.

Incident reporting—Refers to the identification of occurrences that could have led, or did lead, to an undesirable outcome. Reports usually come from personnel directly involved in the incident or events leading up to it (e.g., the nurse, pharmacist, or physician caring for a patient when a medication error occurred) rather than, say, floor managers. From the perspective of those collecting the data, incident reporting counts as a *passive* form of surveillance, relying on those involved in target incidents to provide the desired information. Compared with medical record review and direct observation (*active* methods), incident reporting captures only a fraction of incidents, but has the advantages of relatively low cost and the involvement of frontline personnel in the process of identifying important problems for the organization.

Informed consent— Refers to the process whereby a physician informs a patient about the risks and benefits of a proposed therapy or test, so that the patient can exercise autonomy in deciding whether to proceed. Although the goals of informed consent are irrefutable, consent is often obtained in a haphazard, pro forma fashion, with patients having little true understanding of procedures to which they have consented. Evidence suggests that asking patients to restate the essence of the informed consent improves the quality of these discussions and makes it more likely that the consent is truly "informed."

Just culture—A set of principles that aim to achieve a culture in which frontline personnel feel comfortable disclosing errors—including their own—while maintaining professional accountability. Traditionally, healthcare's culture has held individuals accountable for all errors or mishaps that befall patients under their care. By contrast, a just culture recognizes that individual practitioners should not be held accountable for system failings over which they have no control. A just culture also recognizes many individual or "active" errors represent predictable interactions between human operators and the systems in which they work. However, in contrast to a culture that touts "no blame" as its governing principle, a just culture does not tolerate conscious disregard of clear risks to patients or gross misconduct (e.g., falsifying a record, performing professional duties while intoxicated).

Latent error (or latent condition)—Refers to less apparent failures of organization or design that contributed to the occurrence of errors or allowed them to cause harm to patients. For instance, whereas the active failure in a particular adverse event may have been a mistake in programming an intravenous pump, a latent error might be that the institution uses multiple different types of infusion pumps, making programming errors more likely. Thus, latent errors are quite literally "accidents waiting to happen."

Learning curve—The acquisition of any new skill is associated with the potential for lower-than-expected success rates or higher-than-expected complication rates, a phenomenon known as a "learning curve." While learning curves are almost inevitable when new procedures emerge or new providers are in training, minimizing their impact is a patient safety imperative. One option is to perform initial operations or procedures under the supervision of more experienced operators. Surgical and procedural simulators may play an increasingly important role in decreasing the impact of learning curves on patients, by allowing acquisition of relevant skills in laboratory settings.

Medical Emergency Team—see "Rapid Response Team."

Medication Reconciliation—Patients admitted to a hospital commonly receive new medications or have changes made to their existing medications. As a result, the new medication regimen prescribed at the time of discharge may inadvertently omit needed medications that patients have been receiving for some time. Alternatively, new medications may unintentionally duplicate existing medications. Such unintended inconsistencies in medication regimens may occur at any point of transition in care (e.g., transfer from an intensive care unit [ICU] to a general ward), not just hospital admission or discharge. Medication reconciliation refers to the process of avoiding such inadvertent inconsistencies across transitions in care by reviewing the patient's complete medication regimen at the time of admission, transfer, and discharge and comparing it with the regimen being considered for the new setting of care.

Metacognition—Refers to "thinking about thinking"—that is, reflecting on the thought processes that led to a particular diagnosis or decision to consider whether biases or cognitive short cuts may have had a detrimental effect. Numerous cognitive biases affect human reasoning. In some ways, metacognition amounts to playing devil's advocate with oneself when it comes to working diagnoses and important therapeutic decisions.

Mistakes—In some contexts, errors are dichotomized as "slips" or "mistakes," based on the cognitive psychology of task-oriented behavior. Attentional behavior is characterized by conscious thought, analysis, and planning, as occurs in active problem solving. Schematic behavior refers to the many activities we perform reflexively or as if acting on "autopilot." Complementary to these two behavior types are two categories of error: slips and mistakes. Mistakes reflect failures during attentional behaviors, or incorrect choices. Rather than lapses in concentration (as with slips), mistakes typically involve insufficient knowledge, failure to correctly interpret available information, or application of the wrong cognitive "heuristic" or rule. Thus, choosing the wrong diagnostic test or ordering a suboptimal medication for a given condition represent mistakes. A slip, on the other hand, would be forgetting to check the chart to make sure you ordered them for the right patient.

Near-miss—see "close call."

Normal accident theory—Though less often cited than high reliability theory in the healthcare literature, normal accident theory has played a prominent role in the study of complex organizations. The phrase and theory were developed by sociologist Charles Perrow in connection with a careful analysis of the accident at the Three Mile Island nuclear power plant in 1979 and other industrial (near) catastrophes. In contrast to the optimism of high reliability theory, normal accident theory suggests that, at least in some settings, major accidents become inevitable and, thus, in a sense, "normal." Perrow proposed two factors that create an environment in which a major accident becomes increasingly likely over time: "complexity" and "tight coupling." The degree of complexity envisioned by Perrow occurs when no single operator can immediately foresee the consequences of a given action in the system. Tight coupling occurs when processes are intrinsically time-dependent—once a process has been set in motion, it must be completed within a certain period of time. Many healthcare organizations would illustrate Perrow's definition of complexity, but only hospitals would be regarded as exhibiting tight coupling. Importantly, normal accident theory contends that accidents become inevitable in complex, tightly coupled systems regardless of steps taken to increase safety. In fact, these steps sometimes increase the risk for future accidents through unintended collateral effects and general increases in system complexity.

Normalization of deviance—Term coined by Diane Vaughan in her book *The Challenger Launch Decision: Risky Technology, Culture, and Deviance at NASA*. Vaughn used this expression to describe the gradual shift in what is regarded as normal after repeated exposures to "deviant behavior" (behavior straying from correct [or safe] operating procedure). Corners get cut, safety checks bypassed, and alarms ignored or turned off, and these behaviors become *normal*—not just common, but stripped of their significance as warnings of impending danger.

Patient safety—Freedom from accidental or preventable injuries produced by medical care.

Pay for performance ("P4P")—Refers to the general strategy of promoting quality improvement by rewarding providers (meaning individual clinicians or, more commonly, clinics or hospitals) who meet certain performance expectations with respect to healthcare quality or efficiency. Performance can be defined in terms of patient outcomes but is more commonly defined in terms of processes of care (e.g., the percentage of eligible diabetics who have been referred for annual retinal examinations, or the percentage of patients admitted to the hospital with pneumonia who receive antibiotics within 4 hours).

Plan-Do-Study-Act—Commonly referred to as the PDSA cycle (Figure 3-1), refers to the cycle of activities advocated for achieving process or system improvement. The cycle was first proposed by Walter

Shewhart, one of the pioneers of statistical process control, and popularized by his student, quality expert W. Edwards Deming. The PDSA cycle represents one of the cornerstones of continuous quality improvement (CQI). The components of the cycle are:

- *Plan*: Analyze the problem you intend to improve and devise a plan to correct the problem.

- *Do*: Carry out the plan (preferably as a pilot project to avoid major investments of time or money in unsuccessful efforts).

- *Study*: Did the planned action succeed in solving the problem? If not, what went wrong? If partial success was achieved, how could the plan be refined?

- *Act*: Adopt the change piloted above as is, abandon it as a complete failure, or modify it and run through the cycle again. Regardless of which action is taken, the PDSA cycle continues, either with the same problem or a new one.

Potential ADE—A potential ADE is a medication error or other drug-related mishap that reached the patient but happened not to produce harm (e.g., a penicillin-allergic patient receives penicillin but happens not to have an adverse reaction).

Production pressure—Represents the pressure to put quantity of output—for a product or a service—ahead of safety. This pressure is seen in its starkest form in the "line speed" of factory assembly lines, famously demonstrated by Charlie Chaplin in *Modern Times*, as he is carried away on a conveyor belt and into the giant gears of the factory by the rapidly moving assembly line. In healthcare, production pressure refers to delivery of services—the pressure to run hospitals at 100% capacity, with each bed filled with the sickest possible patients who are discharged at the first sign that they are stable, or the pressure to leave no operating room unused and to keep moving through the schedule for each room as fast as possible. Production pressure produces an organizational culture in which frontline personnel (and often managers as well) are reluctant to suggest any course of action that compromises productivity, even temporarily.

Rapid Response Team (RRT)—The concept of Rapid Response Teams (also known as Medical Emergency Teams) is that of a Code Blue team with more liberal calling criteria. Instead of just frank respiratory or cardiac arrest, RRTs respond to a wide range of worrisome, acute changes in patients' clinical status, such as low blood pressure, difficulty breathing, or altered mental status. In addition to less stringent calling criteria, RRTs (now sometimes called "Rapid Response Systems," to highlight the importance of the activation criteria as well as the response) de-emphasize the traditional hierarchy in patient care in that anyone can initiate the call. Nurses, junior medical staff, or others involved in the care of patients (and, in some hospitals, patients or family members) can call for the assistance of the RRT whenever they are worried about a patient's condition, without having to wait for more senior personnel to assess the patient and approve the decision to call for help.

Read backs—When information is conveyed verbally, miscommunication may occur in a variety of ways, especially when transmission may not occur clearly (e.g., by telephone or radio, or if communication occurs under stress). For names and numbers, the problem often is confusing the sound of one letter or number with another. To address this possibility, the military, civil aviation, and many high-risk industries use protocols for mandatory "read backs," in which the listener repeats the key information, so that the transmitter can confirm its correctness.

Red rules—Rules that must be followed to the letter. In the language of nonhealthcare industries, red rules "stop the line." In other words, any deviation from a red rule will bring work to a halt until compliance is achieved. Red rules, in addition to relating to important and risky processes, must also be simple and easy to remember. An example of a red rule in healthcare might be the following: "No hospitalized patient can undergo a test of any kind, receive a medication or blood product, or undergo a procedure if he or she is not wearing an identification bracelet." Healthcare organizations already have numerous rules and policies that call for strict adherence. So what is it about red rules that makes them more than particularly important rules? The reason that some organizations are using this new designation is that, unlike many standard rules, red rules are ones that will always be supported by the entire organization. In other words, when someone at the front line calls for work to cease on the basis of a red rule, top management must always support this decision.

Root cause analysis—A structured process for identifying the causal or contributing factors underlying adverse events or other critical incidents. The key advantage of RCA over traditional clinical case reviews is that it follows a predefined protocol for identifying specific contributing factors in various causal categories (e.g., personnel, training, equipment, protocols, scheduling) rather than attributing the incident to the first error one finds or to preconceived notions investigators might have about the case.

Rule of thumb—see "heuristic."

Safety culture—Safety culture refers to a commitment to safety that permeates all levels of an organization, from frontline personnel to executive management. More specifically, "safety culture" calls up a number of features identified in studies of HROs, organizations outside of healthcare with exemplary performance with respect to safety, including:

- Acknowledgment of the high-risk, error-prone nature of an organization's activities

- A blame-free environment where individuals are able to report errors or close calls without fear of reprimand or punishment

- An expectation of collaboration across ranks to seek solutions to vulnerabilities

- A willingness on the part of the organization to direct resources to addressing safety concerns

Sentinel event—An adverse event in which death or serious harm to a patient has occurred; usually used to refer to events that are not at all expected or acceptable—for example, an operation on the wrong patient or body part. The choice of the word "sentinel" reflects the egregiousness of the injury (e.g., amputation of the wrong leg) and the likelihood that investigation of such events will reveal serious problems in policies or procedures.

Sensemaking—A term from organizational theory that refers to the processes by which an organization takes in information to make sense of its environment, to generate knowledge, and to make decisions. It is the organizational equivalent of what individuals do when they process information, interpret events in their environments, and make decisions based on these activities.

Sharp end—The "sharp end" refers to the personnel or parts of the healthcare system in direct contact with patients. Personnel operating at the sharp end may literally be holding a scalpel (e.g., an orthopedist who operates on the wrong leg) or figuratively be administering any kind of therapy (e.g., a nurse programming an intravenous pump) or performing any aspect of care. See also "blunt end."

Situational awareness—Refers to the degree to which one's perception of a situation matches reality. In the context of crisis management, where the phrase is most often used, situational awareness includes awareness of fatigue and stress among team members (including oneself), environmental threats to safety, appropriate immediate goals, and the deteriorating status of the crisis (or patient). Failure to maintain situational awareness can result in various problems that compound the crisis. For instance, during a resuscitation, an individual or entire team may focus on a particular task (e.g., a difficult central-line insertion or a particular medication to administer). Fixation on this problem can result in loss of situational awareness to the point that steps are not taken to address immediately life-threatening problems such as respiratory failure or a pulseless rhythm. In this context, maintaining situational awareness might be seen as equivalent to keeping the "big picture" in mind.

Slips (or lapses)—Slips refer to failures of schematic behaviors, or lapses in concentration (e.g., overlooking a step in a routine task as a result of a lapse in memory, an experienced surgeon nicking an adjacent organ during an operation as a result of a momentary lapse in concentration). Mistakes, by contrast, reflect incorrect choices. Distinguishing slips from mistakes serves two important functions. First, the risk factors for their occurrence differ. Slips occur in the face of competing sensory or emotional distractions, fatigue, and stress; mistakes more often reflect lack of experience or insufficient training. Second, the appropriate responses to these error types differ. Reducing the risk of slips requires attention to the designs of protocols, devices, and work environments—using checklists so key steps will not be omitted, reducing fatigue among personnel (or shifting high-risk work away from personnel who have been working extended hours), removing unnecessary variation in the design of key devices, eliminating distractions (e.g., phones) from areas where work requires intense concentration, and other redesign strategies. See also "mistakes."

Standard of care—What the average, prudent clinician would be expected to do under certain circumstances. Standard of care is a term of art in malpractice law, and its definition varies from jurisdiction to jurisdiction. When used in this legal sense, often the standard of care is specific to a given specialty; it is often defined as the care expected of a reasonable practitioner with similar training practicing in the same location under the same circumstances.

Structure-process-outcome triad ("Donabedian Triad")—Quality has been defined as the "degree to which health services for individuals and populations increase the likelihood of desired health outcomes and are consistent with current professional knowledge." This definition, like most others, emphasizes favorable patient outcomes as the gold standard for assessing quality. In practice, however, one would like to detect quality problems without waiting for poor outcomes to develop in such sufficient numbers that deviations from expected rates of morbidity and mortality can be detected. Avedis Donabedian first proposed that quality could be measured using aspects of care (processes or structure) with proven relationships to desirable patient outcomes.

Swiss cheese model—James Reason developed the "Swiss cheese model" (Figure 2–1) to illustrate how analyses of major accidents and catastrophic systems failures tend to reveal multiple, smaller failures leading up to the actual hazard. In the model, each slice of cheese represents a safety barrier or precaution relevant to a particular hazard. For example, if the hazard were wrong-site surgery, slices of cheese might include conventions for identifying siddedness on radiology tests, a protocol for signing the correct site when the surgeon and patient first meet, and a second protocol for reviewing the medical record and checking the previously marked site in the operating room. The point is that no single barrier is foolproof. They each have "holes"; hence, the Swiss cheese. In fact, many of the systems problems discussed by Reason and others—poorly designed work schedules, lack of teamwork, variations in the design of important equipment between and even within institutions—are sufficiently common that many of the slices of cheese already have their holes aligned. In such cases, one slice of cheese may be all that is left between the patient and significant harm.

Systems approach—Medicine has traditionally treated quality problems and errors as failings on the part of individual providers, perhaps reflecting inadequate knowledge or skill levels. The "systems approach," by contrast, takes the view that most errors reflect predictable human failings in the context of poorly designed systems (e.g., expected lapses in human vigilance in the face of long work hours or predictable mistakes on the part of relatively inexperienced personnel faced with cognitively complex situations). Rather than focusing corrective efforts on reprimanding individuals or pursuing remedial education, the systems approach seeks to identify situations or factors likely to give rise to human error and implement "systems changes" that will reduce their occurrence or minimize their impact on patients. This view holds that efforts to catch human errors before they occur or block them from causing harm will ultimately be more fruitful than ones that seek to somehow create flawless providers.

"Time outs"—Refer to planned periods of quiet and/or interdisciplinary discussion focused on ensuring that key procedural details have been addressed. For instance, protocols for ensuring correct site surgery often recommend a "time out" to confirm the identification of the patient, the surgical procedure, site, and other key aspects, often stating them aloud for double-checking by other team members. In addition to avoiding major misidentification errors involving the patient or surgical site, such a time out ensures that all team members share the same "game plan," so to speak.

Triggers—Refer to signals for detecting likely adverse events. For instance, if a hospitalized patient received naloxone (a drug used to reverse the effects of narcotics), the patient probably received an excessive dose of morphine or some other opiate. In this way, triggers can alert patient safety leaders and researchers to probable adverse events so they can review the medical record to determine if an actual or potential adverse event has occurred.

Underuse, overuse, misuse—For process of care, quality problems can arise in one of three ways: underuse, overuse, and misuse. "Underuse" refers to the failure to provide a healthcare service when it would have produced a favorable outcome for a patient. Standard examples include failures to provide appropriate preventive services to eligible patients (e.g., Pap smears, flu shots for elderly patients, screening for hypertension) and proven medications for chronic illnesses (steroid inhalers for asthmatics; aspirin, beta-blockers, and lipid-lowering agents for patients who have suffered a recent myocardial infarction). "Overuse" refers to providing a process of care in circumstances where the potential for harm exceeds the potential for benefit. Prescribing an antibiotic for a viral infection like a cold, for which antibiotics are ineffective, constitutes overuse. "Misuse" occurs when an appropriate process of care has been selected but a preventable complication occurs and the patient does not receive the full potential benefit of the service. Avoidable complications of surgery or medication use are misuse problems. A patient who suffers a rash after receiving penicillin for strep throat, despite having a known allergy to that antibiotic, is an example of misuse. A patient who develops a pneumothorax after an inexperienced operator attempted to insert a subclavian line would represent another example of misuse.

Workaround—From the perspective of frontline personnel trying to accomplish their work, the design of equipment or the policies governing work tasks can seem counterproductive. When frontline personnel adopt consistent patterns of work or ways of bypassing safety features of medical equipment, these patterns and actions are referred to as "workarounds." Although workarounds "fix the problem," the system remains unaltered and thus continues to present potential safety hazards for future patients. From a definitional point of view, it does not matter if frontline users are justified in working around a given policy or equipment design feature. What does matter is that the motivation for a workaround lies in getting work done, not laziness or whim. Thus, the appropriate response by managers to a workaround should not be to reflexively remind staff about the policy and to restate the importance of following it. Rather, workarounds should trigger assessment of workflow and the various competing demands for the time of frontline personnel. In busy clinical areas where efficiency is paramount, managers can expect workarounds to arise whenever policies create added tasks for caregivers, especially when the extra work is out of proportion to the perceived importance of the safety goal.

Reproduced with permission from Shojania KG, Wachter RM. The AHRQ WebM&M glossary. Available at: http://webmm.ahrq.gov/glossary.aspx.

APPENDIX III. SELECTED MILESTONES IN THE FIELD OF PATIENT SAFETY

Year	Event
Fourth century B.C.	Hippocrates writes, "I will never do harm to anyone," which is later translated (and changed) into "Primum non nocere," or "first do no harm."
1857	Ignaz Semmelweiss publishes his findings, demonstrating that hand disinfection leads to fewer infections (puerperal fever).
1863	Florence Nightingale, in *Notes on Hospitals*, writes, "It may seem a strange principle to enunciate as the very first requirement in a Hospital that it should do the sick no harm."
1911	Ernest Codman, a Boston surgeon, establishes his "End Result" hospital—with a goal of following and learning from patient outcomes, include errors in treatment.
1917	The first specialty board (ophthalmology) is formed. Ultimately, 24 boards are founded to certify physicians in the United States.
1918	The American College of Surgeons begins the first program of hospital inspection and certification. In 1951, the program becomes the Joint Commission on Accreditation of Healthcare Organizations (JCAHO), now the Joint Commission.
1959	Robert Moser, an Army physician, publishes *Diseases of Medical Progress*, arguing that iatrogenic disease is common and preventable.

Year	Event
1964	Elihu Schimmel, a Yale physician, publishes one of the first studies of iatrogenic illness, finding that 20% of patients admitted to a university hospital experienced an "untoward episode."
1977	Ivan Illich publishes *Limits of Medicine. Medical Nemesis: the Expropriation of Health*, arguing that healthcare is actually a threat to health.
1985	The Anesthesia Patient Safety Foundation (APSF) is founded, a year after Jeffrey Cooper's seminal paper analyzing failures in anesthesia machines. Twelve years later, the National Patient Safety Foundation is founded, modeled on the APSF.
1990	James Reason publishes *Human Error* (and, 7 years later, *Managing the Risks of Organisational Accidents*), describing his new theory of error as systems failure. His work will go undiscovered by healthcare until Leape's 1994 *JAMA* article.
1991	Publication of Harvard Medical Practice studies (from which the IOM later derives its 44,000–98,000 deaths/year estimate).
1994	Lucian Leape publishes *Error in Medicine* in *JAMA*, the first mainstream article in the healthcare literature arguing for a systems approach to safety.
1999	The release of the IOM report, *To Err is Human*, creates a media sensation and begins the modern patient safety movement.
2000	Following the IOM report, the United Kingdom's National Health Service releases another major report, *An Organisation with a Memory*.
2001	The IOM releases its *Quality Chasm* report.
2001	The Agency for Healthcare Research and Quality (AHRQ) receives 50 million dollars from Congress to begin an aggressive patient safety research and improvement program.
2002	The Joint Commission releases its first National Patient Safety Goals.
2003	The Accreditation Council on Graduate Medical Education institutes duty hours regulations, limiting residents to 80 hours/week.
2004	The U.S. government creates the Office of the National Coordinator for Healthcare IT (ONCHIT), the first federal initiative to computerize healthcare.

Adapted from various sources, particularly Vincent C. *Patient Safety*. London: Elsevier, 2006; and Sharpe VA, Faden AI. *Medical Harm: Historical, Conceptual, and Ethical Dimensions of Iatrogenic Illness*. New York, NY: Cambridge University Press, 1998.

APPENDIX IV. THE JOINT COMMISSION'S NATIONAL PATIENT SAFETY GOALS (HOSPITAL VERSION, 2007)

Goal 1: Improve the accuracy of patient identification.

1A: Use at least two patient identifiers when providing care, treatment, or services.

Goal 2: Improve the effectiveness of communication among caregivers.

2A: For verbal or telephone orders or for telephonic reporting of critical test results, verify the complete order or test result by having the person receiving the information record and "read back" the complete order or test result.

2B: Standardize a list of abbreviations, acronyms, symbols, and dose designations that are not to be used throughout the organization.

2C: Measure, assess and, if appropriate, take action to improve the timeliness of reporting, and the timeliness of receipt by the responsible licensed caregiver, of critical test results and values.

2E: Implement a standardized approach to "hand off" communications, including an opportunity to ask and respond to questions.

Goal 3: Improve the safety of using medications.

3B: Standardize and limit the number of drug concentrations used by the organization.

3C: Identify and, at a minimum, annually review a list of look-alike and sound-alike drugs used by the organization, and take action to prevent errors involving the interchange of these drugs.

3D: Label all medications, medication containers (e.g., syringes, medicine cups, basins), or other solutions on and off the sterile field.

Goal 7: Reduce the risk of healthcare-associated infections.

7A: Comply with current Centers for Disease Control and Prevention (CDC) hand hygiene guidelines.

7B: Manage as sentinel events all identified cases of unanticipated death or major permanent loss of function associated with a healthcare-associated infection.

Goal 8: Accurately and completely reconcile medications across the continuum of care.

8A: There is a process for comparing the patient's current medications with those ordered for the patient while under the care of the organization.

8B: A complete list of the patient's medications is communicated to the next provider of service when a patient is referred or transferred to another setting, service, practitioner, or level of care within or outside the organization. The complete list of medications is also provided to the patient on discharge from the facility.

Goal 9: Reduce the risk of patient harm resulting from falls.

9B: Implement a fall reduction program including an evaluation of the effectiveness of the program.

Goal 13: Encourage patients' active involvement in their own care as a patient safety strategy.

13A: Define and communicate the means for patients and their families to report concerns about safety and encourage them to do so.

Goal 15: The organization identifies safety risks inherent in its patient population.

15A: The organization identifies patients at risk for suicide. (Applicable to psychiatric hospitals and patients being treated for emotional or behavioral disorders in general hospitals.)

Reproduced with permission from http://www.jointcommission.org/PatientSafety/NationalPatientSafetyGoals/07_hap_cah_npsgs.htm.

Skipped numbers represent retired Goals (the numbers are not replaced).

APPENDIX V. AGENCY FOR HEALTHCARE RESEARCH AND QUALITY'S (AHRQ) PATIENT SAFETY INDICATORS (PSIs)

Hospital-level Patient Safety Indicators (20 indicators)

- Complications of anesthesia (PSI 1)
- Death in low mortality DRGs (PSI 2)
- Decubitus ulcer (PSI 3)
- Failure to rescue (PSI 4)
- Foreign body left in during procedure (PSI 5)
- Iatrogenic pneumothorax (PSI 6)
- Selected infections due to medical care (PSI 7)
- Postoperative hip fracture (PSI 8)
- Postoperative hemorrhage or hematoma (PSI 9)
- Postoperative physiologic and metabolic derangements (PSI 10)
- Postoperative respiratory failure (PSI 11)
- Postoperative pulmonary embolism or DVT (PSI 12)
- Postoperative sepsis (PSI 13)

- Postoperative wound dehiscence in abdominopelvic surgical patients (PSI 14)
- Accidental puncture and laceration (PSI 15)
- Transfusion reaction (PSI 16)
- Birth trauma—injury to neonate (PSI 17)
- Obstetric trauma—vaginal delivery with instrument (PSI 18)
- Obstetric trauma—vaginal delivery without instrument (PSI 19)
- Obstetric trauma—cesarean delivery (PSI 20)

Area-level patient safety indicators (7 indicators)

- Foreign body left in during procedure (PSI 21)
- Iatrogenic pneumothorax (PSI 22)
- Selected infections due to medical care (PSI 23)
- Postoperative wound dehiscence in abdominopelvic surgical patients (PSI 24)
- Accidental puncture and laceration (PSI 25)
- Transfusion reaction (PSI 26)
- Postoperative hemorrhage or hematoma (PSI 27)

Reproduced with permission from Patient Safety Indicators Overview. AHRQ Quality Indicators. Rockville, MD: Agency for Healthcare Research and Quality, February 2006. Available at: http://www.qualityindicators.ahrq.gov/psi_overview.htm.

APPENDIX VI. THE NATIONAL QUALITY FORUM'S LIST OF 28 "NEVER EVENTS"

Surgical events

- Surgery performed on the wrong body part
- Surgery performed on the wrong patient
- Wrong surgical procedure performed on a patient
- Unintended retention of a foreign object in a patient after surgery or other procedure

- Intraoperative or immediately postoperative death in an American Society of Anesthesiologists (ASA) Class I patient

Care management events

- Patient death or serious disability associated with a medication error (e.g., errors involving the wrong drug, wrong dose, wrong patient, wrong time, wrong rate, wrong preparation, or wrong route of administration)
- Patient death or serious disability associated with a hemolytic reaction caused by the administration of ABO/HLA-incompatible blood or blood products
- Maternal death or serious disability associated with labor or delivery in a low-risk pregnancy while being cared for in a healthcare facility
- Patient death or serious disability associated with hypoglycemia, the onset of which occurs while the patient is being cared for in a healthcare facility
- Death or serious disability (kernicterus) associated with failure to identify and treat hyperbilirubinemia in neonates
- Stage 3 or 4 pressure ulcers acquired after admission to a healthcare facility
- Patient death or serious disability caused by spinal manipulative therapy
- Artificial insemination with the wrong donor sperm or donor egg

Product or device events

- Patient death or serious disability associated with the use of contaminated drugs, devices, or biologics provided by the healthcare facility
- Patient death or serious disability associated with the use or function of a device in patient care, in which the device is used or functions other than as intended
- Patient death or serious disability associated with intravascular air embolism that occurs while being cared for in a healthcare facility

Environmental events

- Patient death or serious disability associated with an electric shock or elective cardioversion while being cared for in a healthcare facility
- Any incident in which a line designated for oxygen or other gas to be delivered to a patient contains the wrong gas or is contaminated by toxic substances
- Patient death or serious disability associated with a burn incurred from any source while being cared for in a healthcare facility
- Patient death or serious disability associated with the use of restraints or bedrails while being cared for in a healthcare facility
- Patient death or serious disability associated with a fall while being cared for in a healthcare facility

Patient protection events

- Infant discharged to the wrong person
- Patient death or serious disability associated with patient elopement (disappearance)
- Patient suicide, or attempted suicide resulting in serious disability, while being cared for in a healthcare facility

Criminal events

- Any instance of care ordered by or provided by someone impersonating a physician, nurse, pharmacist, or other licensed healthcare provider
- Abduction of a patient of any age
- Sexual assault on a patient within or on the grounds of the healthcare facility
- Death or significant injury of a patient or staff member resulting from a physical assault (i.e., battery) that occurs within or on the grounds of the healthcare facility

APPENDIX VII. THINGS PATIENTS AND FAMILIES CAN DO, AND QUESTIONS THEY CAN ASK, TO IMPROVE THEIR CHANCES OF REMAINING SAFE IN THE HOSPITAL

Things to Do to Prevent Errors in a Hospital or Nursing Home

What to do or check	Discussion or recommendation
Make friends with your nurses, phlebotomists, and other hospital personnel. Make sure they address you by name at least once each shift.	
Before you are given a medication, ask what it is and what it's for.	
Before you are given a medication, a transfusion, an x-ray, or a procedure, make sure the nurse confirms your name both by asking you and checking your wristband.	A few hospitals may supplement this through the use of bar coding; for example, checking that the bar code on your wristband and the bar code on a medication bottle match.
Before being taken off the floor for a procedure, ask what it is and be sure you understand where you are going and why.	
Be sure your family members' contact information is available to the hospital or nursing home personnel.	It is not a bad idea to place a card with your family members' contact information by your bedside (in addition to being sure that this information is in the chart).
Before being transferred from floor-to-floor in a hospital (such as from the ICU to the general medical or surgical floor) or from one institution to another, check to be sure all catheters and other paraphernalia that should be removed have been.	Sometimes (particularly when there are no checklists), caregivers will forget to remove an IV line or urinary catheter before a transfer, which creates an unnecessary risk of infections. Believe it or not, doctors (one out of three in one study) will often forget whether their patient even has a urinary catheter in place. Don't be reluctant to ask your doctors or nurses whether you still need your catheters after the urgent need for them has passed.

What to do or check	Discussion or recommendation
Ask your caregivers whether they have washed (or cleaned) their hands.	Increasingly, you won't see them wash their hands, because they will be rubbing their hands with an antiseptic hand-gel placed in a dispenser outside your room. This gel appears to provide better protection against infection than routine handwashing.
If you have an Advance Directive (and you should), keep a copy with you, make sure your family has one, give one to your nurse or doctor to place on your chart, and be certain it is transferred from site to site with you.	

Being an Informed Consumer: Patient Safety Questions for the Hospital's Patient Safety or Quality Departments

What to do or check	Discussion or recommendation
Does the hospital have CPOE, an electronic medical record, and bar coding? If not, when do they plan to have them?	It would be great if they had them and they were up and running. If they have CPOE, ask what percent of physicians' orders are written on the computerized system (if it is less than half, then the docs are still kicking the tires and the system is not really implemented). If CPOE and bar coding are not in place (fewer than 20% of hospitals presently have them), it should be budgeted to be in place within 3–5 years. If not, I'd worry.
Is there a functioning, preferably computerized, incident reporting system, on which hospital personnel can report errors and near-misses?	The computerized systems make reporting, and dissemination of the information, much easier. So it would be good to hear, "yes we do."
How many incident reports are logged each month?	Although it might seem counterintuitive, the more the better. If a midsized hospital (300 or so beds) doesn't receive at least 100 reports a month,

What to do or check	Discussion or recommendation
	then I'd worry that the hospital lacks a reporting culture: workers aren't sharing errors and near-misses either because they are worried about blame or they are convinced that it isn't worth reporting because reports enter a black hole.
What is done with these reports?	You'd like to know that they go to the relevant managers in the area (the catheterization lab, the OR), who are expected to respond to them. Also, there should be an uber-manager who watches for trends (e.g., an uptick in patient falls, bed ulcers, or medication administration errors).
How many detailed root cause analyses have been done in the past year?	Like the incident reports, you might think that "zero" would be a great answer because it would mean there were no major errors. But you can be sure that there were. So I'd expect that the average hospital will have done at least 10 full-blown RCAs in the past year.
Is there a Patient Safety Officer who is compensated for this role? What are his or her qualifications?	Many hospitals will not have a paid Patient Safety Officer yet, but all midsize and large hospitals should have one in the next few years. This guarantees that it is someone's job to be concerned about safety. It should be a respected physician, nurse, or pharmacist with additional training in human factors, systems engineering, quality improvement, and similar areas.
Is there an active Patient Safety Committee that meets at least monthly?	The answer must be yes.
Are there trained intensivists in the critical care units (ICUs) and hospitalists on the medical wards?	There is strong evidence that the on-site presence of intensivists, at least during the day, is associated with better ICU outcomes. For small hospitals without intensivists, linking the ICU electronically to trained intensivists who remotely monitor the patients also seems to improve outcomes. The evidence supporting the value of hospitalists caring for general medical

What to do or check	Discussion or recommendation
	and surgical patients is not quite as strong, but two studies did show lower death rates. I believe that the on-site presence of physicians who specialize in overseeing and coordinating patients' hospital care is likely to improve safety.
Are the physicians who will care for you board certified in their specialty?	All else being equal, board certification indicates that your physician has demonstrated a certain level of knowledge and competence.
What is the nurse-to-patient ratio, and what percentage of the nurses are registered nurses (RNs)?	Ratios of more than 6–7 to 1 on the medical and surgical wards are associated with higher rates of errors (it should be much lower, like 2 to 1, in the ICUs). Error rates also seem to be higher when more than about 30% of total nursing care is delivered by non-RNs (i.e., licensed practical nurses or nurses' aides).
Are there clinical pharmacists on the hospital wards who can help you understand and organize your medications?	There is good evidence that the involvement of clinical pharmacists, particularly in the discharge process, improves safety.
Does the hospital run simulator or other specific teamwork training?	Ideally, the hospital would require simulator training for people working in high-risk areas like the OR, ER, and on Code Blue teams. In addition, specific teamwork training (CRM) is probably helpful, and a hospital that has an organized simulator and CRM program is probably ahead of the patient safety curve.
What does the hospital do to prevent handoff errors?	We would want to know that, at very least, there are read backs of verbal orders and checklists before patients move from one unit to another (like the ICU to the floor or from the floor to a nursing home).
What patient safety initiatives has the hospital undertaken in the past year?	They should have at least one or two that they can describe proudly, preferably with measurable results they can cite.

Index